PRINCIPLES OF PROFESSIONAL STUDIES IN NURSING

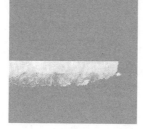

Principles of Professional Studies in Nursing

Edited by

Janice Brown and Paula Libberton

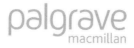

palgrave
macmillan

First published 2007 by
PALGRAVE MACMILLAN
Houndmills, Basingstoke, Hampshire RG21 6XS and
175 Fifth Avenue, New York, N.Y. 10010
Companies and representatives throughout the world

PALGRAVE MACMILLAN is the global academic imprint of the Palgrave
Macmillan division of St. Martin's Press, LLC and of Palgrave Macmillan Ltd.
Macmillan® is a registered trademark in the United States, United Kingdom
and other countries. Palgrave is a registered trademark in the European
Union and other countries.

ISBN-13: 978–1–4039–4223–4
ISBN-10: 1–4039–4223–4

This book is printed on paper suitable for recycling and made from fully
managed and sustained forest sources.

A catalogue record for this book is available from the British Library.

10   9   8   7   6   5   4   3   2   1
16   15   14   13   12   11   10   09   08   07

Printed and bound in China

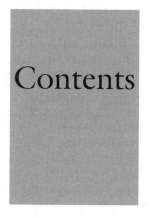

Contents

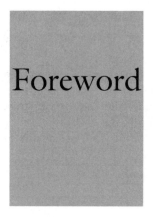

Foreword

It is my great pleasure to write the Foreword for this important new book. The aspirations of the authors are high and every student of nursing ought to use this volume as the map by which to plot a successful nursing career. Embedded in each chapter are the fundamental principles that surround nursing and caring; those elements that help us to navigate the complexities of patient-centred care. Committing ourselves to exploring such concepts as the ethics of caring, spirituality, nursing theory and evidence-based practice is vital in a health care world that is constantly changing.

As I reflect upon the principles that are most important for those students who have chosen to entrust their skills, intellect, energy and talent to the honourable discipline of nursing, I am reminded of a story recounted to me by a colleague. Her mother, who suffered from Alzheimer's disease, had been admitted to a medical ward in a local hospital for routine tests. One evening my colleague visited her mother to find her in a very agitated state. The patient opposite her mother had died and the deceased patient's relatives – who were very religious – were holding a vigil by the bedside, singing hymns and praying. As a consequence, my colleague's mother believed she was attending her own funeral and became very upset and anxious. It took her daughter and staff a significant period of time to calm her and the whole incident was very traumatic for all involved.

This incident provokes a number of questions, the range of which underlines the diverse principles and concepts involved in the practical business of nursing care. Could the situation have been avoided? Did it matter that an old confused woman and her daughter were unnecessarily upset? If so, whose responsibility was it to ensure that the environment of care was compatible with the needs of the patients and their relatives? What were the moral dilemmas faced by the different actors in the story? What organisational and systems issues arose? Who could and should have made an assessment of the changing needs of my colleague's mother as the event around her unfolded? How could the management of either patient have been justified in terms of ethics, common sense, evidence-based practice or basic humanity? How do nurses find themselves in compromised situations where they are having to defend situations that cause unnecessary suffering and anxiety?

Such dilemmas are the mainstay of everyday nursing practice. This book helps to outline the basic principles by which each one of us can begin to chart our professional path through the delivery of patient-centred nursing care. By identifying and reflecting upon the issues the book contains, we become better equipped to make decisions when confronted with difficult scenarios in our work as nurses. Enjoy and embrace the challenges!

Alison Kitson, PhD, RN, FRCN
Executive Director, Nursing
Royal College of Nursing
August 2006

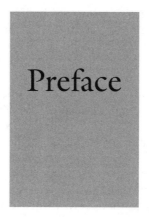

Preface

Principles of Professional Studies in Nursing aims to support you, as a student of nursing, to strive for excellence in patient-centred care; to practise with self-awareness, compassion, confidence and competence to high ethical and clinical standards from a sound knowledge base; and to be cognisant, creative and proactive to policy, research and a range of evidence to secure the respect and confidence of the people you serve. This is challenging, but equipped with an openness of mind and a thirst for knowledge, you should be able to enjoy the journey.

The topics addressed in this book range from the nature and history of nursing, humanities for nursing, ethics, reflection, spirituality, nursing theory, policy, quality assurance, clinical governance, leadership and evidence-based practice. These areas of knowledge can be considered difficult to grasp as they are conceptually rich and quite different from the traditional subjects of anatomy, physiology and pharmacology. However, bringing them together in one text offers you the opportunity to develop and extend your knowledge base of professional issues in nursing.

The elements of a typical UK undergraduate nursing programme exist to prepare you to designated standards of proficiency and education for practice (NMC 2004a). Your programme should incorporate the practice experience, the study of life sciences and the study of psychology and sociology, collectively known as the social sciences. However, there are also other essential elements important to emerging practitioners of nursing, such as an understanding of the nature and theories of nursing, applied ethics, reflection for practice, the importance of spirituality, consideration of policy, quality assurance, leadership and evidence-based practice. These essential issues are concerned with the complexities of nursing: its ways of being; its quest for effective and quality care delivery; and the importance of getting the right care, based on the best evidence available. Although the heart of nursing is rooted in these issues, two problems arise. The first is the vagueness of an umbrella nomenclature or classification term uniting these issues, and the second is the absence of a key introductory text. Different institutions approach these issues in different ways but in response to the consistent student demand in Southampton, this book was developed to portray and discuss the principles of professional studies in nursing.

It has been written by a range of talented contributors who have a passion for excellence in nursing and have addressed; the need for a philosophy of care; the knowledge and application of leadership and management skills; and the skill and ability to integrate appropriate evidence for clinical practice. These three areas are used as the organising framework for the book but they are so interlinked that although their division allows for individual attention and structure, you will appreciate they are entwined components for professional practice. The contributors refer to each other's work across chapters and sections as the principles of professional studies are revealed as a complex matrix of values and knowledge.

Each chapter begins with a list of contents and learning outcomes so you can gain a sense of the issues being addressed. Throughout, there are activities which you are invited to complete. These activities have been designed to further your understanding and application of the issues being discussed and are an important part of achieving the stated learning outcomes. Please do take the time to engage with them, either on your own, with a colleague or a group of fellow students so you can reflect on your own values for practice, its context, your personal and professional knowledge development and your nursing contribution to people who need nursing intervention. At the end of each chapter you will find self-evaluation questions to challenge your understanding and developing knowledge base.

You may find that you like to visit particular individual chapters or that you prefer to read the complete text in order. Either way, the most important thing is that you use it to meet your needs and learning style.

Part I is the largest part of the book, consisting of Chapters 1–6. This part is called Principles within Nursing as it is concerned with supporting you to appreciate knowledge, values and beliefs which guide your practice. In this part you are encouraged to explore the history and nature of nursing; to consider your own values for living and being part of nursing; to appreciate and understand the contribution of nursing theory to this emerging discipline; and to examine the purpose and process of reflection. You can read about ethical ways of knowing and making judgements in complex situations. You are invited to appreciate the meaning of illness and suffering through considering how poetry, music and literature can enhance your understanding of illness experiences. Finally, but importantly, you are invited to consider whole person care through the human dimension of spirituality.

In Part II the focus is on the Management of Care, which is concerned with understanding the external influences and the skills necessary in care delivery. Chapters 7–9 focus on the impact of policy of nursing care and state the importance for nurses to have an understanding of policy and policy development at local and national level to be proactive in influencing the health agenda. Linked to policy is a chapter on quality and clinical governance, important principles in the health care agenda of the twenty-first century. Management and leadership in health care are inextricably linked, so the final chapter in this section examines leadership through presenting definitions, qualities, leadership theories and theories of motivation. It concludes with exercises on how to examine yourself in terms of your readiness for and effectiveness in leadership for practice.

The final Part III consists of Chapters 10–12, which focus on evidence-based practice, clinical effectiveness and knowledge management. You are introduced to the concept of evidence-based practice and its relationship to clinical effectiveness. The issue of values arises again but this time in the context of research paradigms. Hierarchies of evidence are explained and considered in the context of how they have generated tension in the argument regarding, 'what is the best evidence for practice-based problems?'. You are introduced to skills that support you to seek the best available evidence, on how to think critically and how to critically appraise evidence for application in practice. The concluding chapter affirms the relevance and importance of professional studies and the complexities of practice, whilst appreciating the legacies of the development of nursing and its future course. It is suggested how the application of knowledge to practice is dependent not only on the right knowledge but also on the calibre of nurses to be able to lead and manage care skilfully within a changing health and social care context. Developing communities of practice and knowledge networks are suggested as ways of making the integration of evidence into practice more effective.

We hope this preface has motivated you to read further. We are confident you will find this book interesting, challenging and informative to support your knowledge and practice within the principles of professional nursing.

Janice Brown
Paula Libberton

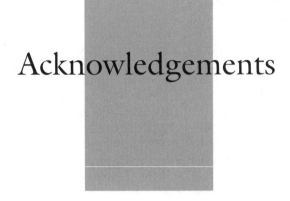

Acknowledgements

Janice Brown and Paula Libberton would like to acknowledge the enthusiasm and commitment of the students of the School of Nursing and Midwifery, University of Southampton, for setting the challenge of writing this book to support their study and practice of Professional Studies in Nursing.

Rob Carter, the author of Chapter 8: Quality and Clinical Governance, wishes to acknowledge the important advice and contributions he received from Jane Cant, Clinical Risk Manager, Southampton University Hospitals NHS Trust; David Ferguson, Consultant Nurse (Mental Health in Learning Disability), Hampshire Partnership NHS Trust; and Patricia Radway, Clinical Governance Manager, Hampshire Partnership NHS Trust.

Notes on Contributors

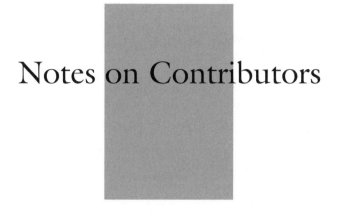

Chris Bailey is Lecturer in Nursing and Academic Lead for the Cancer, Palliative and End of Life Care academic development group in the School of Nursing and Midwifery, University of Southampton.

Janice Brown is Senior Lecturer in Nursing, a Health Foundation post-doctoral fellow, and a member of the Cancer, Palliative and End of Life Care research group in the School of Nursing and Midwifery, University of Southampton.

Rob Carter is Lecturer and a member of the Public Health (First Point of Contact and Public Protection) academic development group in the School of Nursing and Midwifery, University of Southampton.

Yvette Cox is Lecturer in Nursing, Award Leader for the BSc (Hons) and Diploma in Health Care Studies and a member of the Public Health (First Point of Contact and Public Protection) academic development group in the School of Nursing and Midwifery, University of Southampton.

Mary Gobbi is Senior Lecturer in Nursing, Award Leader for the Post-graduate Diploma/RN programme and a member of the High Dependency academic development group in the School of Nursing and Midwifery, University of Southampton. Mary also co-ordinates the nursing group in the EU Commission Tuning Project, which is developing common reference competences across different disciplines.

Lorraine Ireland is Lecturer in Nursing and a member of the Family and Child academic development group in the School of Nursing and Midwifery, University of Southampton.

Andrée le May is Professor of Nursing, Award Lead for the Clinical Doctoral programme and Academic Lead for the Public Health (First Point of Contact and Public Protection) academic development group in the School of Nursing and Midwifery, University of Southampton.

Paula Libberton is Lecturer in Nursing and a member of the Mental Health academic development group in the School of Nursing and Midwifery, University of Southampton.

Sian Maslin-Prothero is Professor of Nursing in the School of Nursing and Midwifery, Keele University.

Peter Savage is Lecturer in Nursing and a member of the Mental Health academic development group in the School of Nursing and Midwifery, University of Southampton.

Sue Toward is Lecturer and a member of the Public Health (First Point of Contact and Public Protection) academic development group in the School of Nursing and Midwifery, University of Southampton.

Pauline Turner is Lecturer in Nursing, Award Leader for the BSc (Hons) Clinical Practice and a member of the Cancer, Palliative and End of Life Care academic development group in the School of Nursing and Midwifery, University of Southampton.

Principles Within Nursing

1

Introduction to Professional Studies in Nursing

Janice Brown and Mary Gobbi

CONTENTS

■ The nature of nursing

■ Values

■ NMC code of conduct (NMC 2004b)

■ Knowledge used in nursing

■ Historical landmarks in nursing

LEARNING OUTCOMES

This chapter should enable you to

■ Appreciate debates about the nature of nursing

■ Explore the meaning and significance of values in nursing, of self and others

■ Appreciate how different types of knowledge support the practice and discipline of nursing

■ Be aware of the interface of nursing in relation to other health care professions

■ Identify historical landmarks in the development of nursing in the United Kingdom

1.1 Introduction

As the focus of this book is to support your education as a student nurse, it is not only useful to begin by identifying the principles of professional nursing but also to consider their history, epistemology (knowledge foundations), values (or sense of being, their ontology) and more pragmatically, what sort of occupation nursing is or claims to be.

Note the term 'occupation' was used when describing nursing in the above paragraph and not 'profession' as, according to sociologically defined criteria (Whittington and Boore 1988), nursing is not classified as a profession in the same sense as medicine and law. The United Kingdom Standard Occupational Classification (2000) system (see Box 1.1), organised by the government agency of the Office of National Statistics (ONS), classifies nursing in the third major occupational group entitled 'Associate professional and technical occupations'. Other therapists like physiotherapists, occupational therapists, and speech and language therapists are also classified in this third major group. This recognition of being associate professionals is interesting and may account for the common usage of the term 'nursing profession' as an identifying label for the body of people who are registered nurses in the United Kingdom. However, nursing is also considered a practice-based discipline, as its actions are rooted in practice and it is considered an 'emerging discipline' in universities, which means it is in the process of establishing its knowledge and evidence base. Therefore nursing, and its therapist partners, is in transition both in occupational and academic status.

BOX 1.1 Standard occupational classification (2000)

Major groups

1. Managers and senior officials

2. Professional occupations

3. Associate professional and technical occupations

4. Administrative and secretarial occupations

5. Skilled trades occupations

6. Personal service occupations

7. Sales and customer service occupations

8. Process, plant and machine operatives

9. Elementary occupations

Source: National statistics website: (http://www.statistics.gov.uk. Crown copyright material is reproduced with the permission to the controller of HMSO).

Nursing also has a long tradition of being identified as a vocation, with aspirations of being a profession. The sense of vocation appears to originate from its roots in caring and service to others, as exemplified by Florence Nightingale. The idea of nursing as a profession, in the United Kingdom, lies at the door of the nursing pioneer, Mrs Bedford Fenwick, who fought for registration and legal protection of the title 'registered nurse'. These ideas of vocation and profession sit in tension, even today. Vocation has not only the positive connotation of service to others and altruism but also negative suggestions of subservience and obedience. The term 'profession' initially appears an honourable aspiration through the assumption that it possesses a distinct body of knowledge and self-regulates but profession has its negative side as well with associations of power, superiority and exclusivity. Therefore, neither the term 'vocation' nor 'profession' seem entirely helpful for supporting the image of a group of people whose goals are to promote effective patient-centred care through drawing on up-to-date evidence and who are accountable for their practice. However, this indelible mix presents a cultural and historical legacy to nursing which is reflected across much of the world (Cameron-Traub 1991).

When thinking about the term 'professionalism', our understanding is that registered nurses should aspire to achieve excellence in patient-centred care; to practice with awareness, compassion and competence to high ethical and clinical standards from an up-to-date knowledge base; and to be cognisant, proactive and responsive to policy, research and knowledge generation to merit the respect and confidence of the people they serve. It could be argued that the other therapist professions are of a similar mind, particularly as the drive for inter-professional co-operation in learning, practice and knowledge generation is central to health and social care in the twenty-first century. This meaning of 'professionalism' is what we aspire to promote and explore in this text, to offer you, as students of nursing, the opportunity to understand and consider your own contribution to professional practice.

In this chapter we begin our journey of exploring these principles which raise many questions for us to consider: What is nursing? What are its values and its knowledge base? What are the origins of nursing? These important questions often become neglected in the quest for pursuing contemporary professional nursing but they are important to consider because they can help us in our understanding of nursing and its particular contribution to society and offer clues for its future direction. Let us begin our journey.

1.2 What is nursing?

The history and diversity of nursing is reflected in the people who might consider themselves 'nurses'. Some nurses hold the legally protected title of registered nurse (RN) following successful completion of a recognised education programme, when their name is entered onto the Nursing and Midwifery Council (NMC) Register. This register became a legal requirement only in 1919 in the United Kingdom when the first State Registered Nurse (SRN) entry was Mrs Bedford Fenwick. Today, it holds the names of a range of 'registered nurse' titles including adult nurses, sick children's nurses, specialist community public health nurses, mental health nurses and learning disability nurses. This registration qualification used to be gained on its own through successful completion of a hospital-based nurse training programme but since 1989 (UKCC 1986) academic qualifications have been entwined with the statutory requirement. Thereafter, additional qualifications and awards can be sought from a range of awarding bodies. The body of registered nurses (approx 670,000 in United Kingdom today as compared to 70,000 in 1901) may also hold an array of role descriptors, illustrating their additional skills and responsibilities such as research nurse, clinical nurse specialist, matron and consultant nurse.

So what kind of 'occupation' is nursing? What do nurses do (nursing actions), what kinds of knowledge do nurses create or draw upon in practice and research and what might nurses be and do in the future? Look at Activity 1.1 and consider your responses to the questions posed.

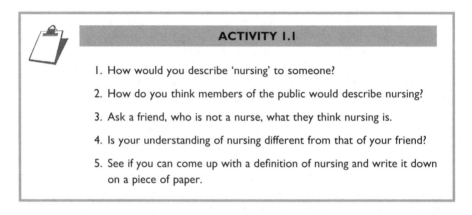

ACTIVITY 1.1

1. How would you describe 'nursing' to someone?

2. How do you think members of the public would describe nursing?

3. Ask a friend, who is not a nurse, what they think nursing is.

4. Is your understanding of nursing different from that of your friend?

5. See if you can come up with a definition of nursing and write it down on a piece of paper.

Contemporary nursing in the United Kingdom and Europe has evolved over many centuries in response to the social, economic and political challenges of its time. First, we will consider nursing in the context of 'today' before looking into the past.

1.3 Nursing today

Nursing is practised in a range of settings inclusive of acute trusts (hospitals), primary care trusts (patients' homes and community hospitals), prisons and special authorities. A commonality of all the settings is for registered practitioners to be on a register which in the United Kingdom is the NMC register. The main functions of the NMC are to protect the public. It promotes this by setting professional standards for registration through the Code of Professional Conduct (NMC 2004b) and having powers to remove practitioners from its register if they contravene the fitness for practice rule (Statutory Instrument 2004/1761).

The essential standards of proficiency (previously known as competencies) for pre-registration nursing education have been written by the NMC in line with the Nursing and Midwifery Order 2001 (Statutory Instrument 2004/254). There are 17 proficiency standards which must be achieved 'in the context of practice in their chosen branch' (NMC 2004a: 22), be it adult nursing, mental health nursing, learning disabilities nursing or children's nursing. These proficiency standards are the bedrock of current first-level nurse education programmes in the United Kingdom and you will probably most readily see them in some form in your practice documents, where they may be assessed as competencies or standards. You can access them in full from the NMC website (www.nmc-uk.org). The educational standard is set at a minimum level of a diploma of higher education, although there are also direct entry programmes which are set at undergraduate and master's level. Increasingly, other countries have already moved to an all-graduate profession of nursing (e.g. Ireland, Scotland, Wales and Australia) but this is still a point for political, economic and cultural tension in England.

The practice of nursing and the role of nurses are clearly influenced by government policy, which has been prolific in the United Kingdom over the last 10 years (see Chapter 7). A particular policy of note is the 'The New NHS: Modern and Dependable' (DoH 1999a), which made it clear that Trusts would be expected to strengthen the nursing, midwifery and health visiting contribution to health and health care and make a commitment to consult a new strategy for nursing, midwifery and health visiting. 'Making a Difference' (DoH 1999b) sets out the government's strategic intentions for nursing, midwifery and health visiting for the coming years, indicating plans to expand the workforce; strengthen education and training; develop a modern career framework; improve working lives; enhance quality; strengthen leadership; modernise professional self-regulation; and encourage and support new roles and new ways of working. The Wanless Report (2002) analysed the historical patterns and a few trends in health and social care, identifying the likely health care needs of the future (see Chapter 7). Balanced against these trends was the current and predicted shortage of nurses, midwives and other health care professionals, which is a worldwide issue. The Report clearly argued for changes in the way services are delivered and the way practitioners need to work. The Department of Health websites offer clear examples of nursing initiatives in caring and supporting people in new roles and in new ways; for example, the guidance document entitled 'Supporting people with long term conditions: liberating the talents of nurses who care for people with long term conditions' (see www.dh.gov.uk/publications).

The Knowledge and Skills Framework (KSF) (DoH 2004a) defines and describes the knowledge and skills which qualified and registered NHS staff (including nurses) need to apply in order to deliver quality services. This also lies at the heart of career and pay progression, linked into life-long learning and the new pay process called 'Agenda for Change' (DoH 2004b). These initiatives have been met with excitement and optimism in the sense that it is perceived that nursing is valued by the state and supported by investment. However, issues of limited leadership in nursing, the lack of a coherent career structure and the quest but inability to define itself also gives it a sense of tension.

Increasingly, international and European influences are also growing in the practice, regulation and definition of nursing. The International Labour Organisation (ILO 1977) identifies three levels of nursing personnel. Despite sociological and UK government statistical classification of nursing as not being a full profession, the international first level is called the *professional nurse*, which is the registered nurse and is described as someone who has the education and training 'recognised as necessary for assuming highly complex and respons-ible functions and authorised to perform them'. Although the title 'registered nurse' is protected in English law, this is not consistent throughout the world. However, the International Council of Nursing (1998) argued that the title of 'nurse' should be legally protected and used only by those legally author-ised to provide the full scope of nursing. They considered that this scope of nursing practice includes the following spheres of responsibility: giving direct care; supervising others; leading; managing; teaching; undertaking research; and developing health policy for health care systems (ICN 1998).

The importance of being able to define nursing was supported by the Royal College of Nursing (RCN) in 2003. In their document 'Defining Nursing' (RCN 2003), they cite a government department which suggests the major responsibilities of each professional group are quite clear, with the exception of nursing. They also cite an economist who indicates that nursing is vulnerable to inappropriate use without such clarity. Removing this lack of clarity has been championed by many nurses with an original but dated definition of nursing from Virginia Henderson in the 1960s:

> The unique function of the nurse is to assist the individual, sick or well, in the performance of those activities contributing to health or its recovery (or to peaceful death) that he would perform unaided if he had the necessary strength, will, or knowledge. And to do this in such as way as to help him gain independence as rapidly as possible . . .
>
> (Henderson 1991: 21)

This definition is still widely used across the world. It does continue to distin-guish between the independent aspect of nursing (which is the part cited) and the interdependent aspect where medicine and other health care team members are indicated, which is 'critical to understanding the complexity of nursing and its particular contribution within the multi-disciplinary team' (RCN 2003: 7).

Another American definition of the 1980s cites, 'nursing is the diagnosis and treatment of human responses to actual or potential threats to health' (ANA 1980), which is important in that it focuses on human responses in the context of health rather than disease.

The RCN distinguishes between professional nursing and the nursing under-taken by other people as it claims that,

> The distinction between professional nursing and the nursing undertaken by other persons does not lie in the task performed, nor in the level of skill that is required to perform a particular task; as for professional practice, the difference lies in:

> - The knowledge that is the basis of the assessment of need and the determination of the action to meet the need
>
> - The clinical judgement inherent in the processes of assessment, diagnosis, prescription and evaluation

- The personal accountability for all decisions and actions, including the decision to delegate to others

- The structured relationship between the nurse and the patient which incorporates professional regulation and a code of ethics within a statutory framework.

(RCN 2003: 4)

The RCN document concludes with its definition that nursing is 'The use of clinical judgement in the provision of care to enable people to improve, maintain, or recover health to cope with health problems, and to achieve the best possible quality of life, whatever their disability, until death' (RCN 2003: 3). This is then supported by six defining characteristics. Have a look at Activity 1.2 to help you explore this document in more detail.

ACTIVITY 1.2

What are the main distinctions between the RCN (2003) definition and that of Virginia Henderson (1991)?

See if you can find three definitions of nursing in the literature. Write them down and compare them.

Access and read the Royal College of Nursing's document 'Defining Nursing' (RCN 2003) on www.rcn.org.uk. It contains many definitions of nursing and offers a discussion about how different countries have defined it.

How do these definitions compare with your description of nursing from Activity 1.1?
Why do you think it is so difficult to define nursing?
Do you think it is important to define nursing?

Whatever definition of nursing is supported, most nurses would agree that nursing involves a relationship between the nurse, another person, the general public, the meaning of health, the environment and society, hence nursing philosophy (examining the beliefs and values held by nursing in relation to these concepts) has to address these issues and what we understand by them. Nursing theory and nursing models are discussed in Chapter 2. These are often considered to be a knowledge base for nurses, which draw on a range of knowledge from other disciplines but can also be used as a guide for practice.

There are propositions in the literature, often espoused as nursing theory, that nursing is relational (Peplau 1952), and involves caring (Watson 1985) and particular ways of being and doing (Paterson and Zderad 1976). Nursing is a person-based occupation, generally acknowledged to be both an art and a science (Kitson 1993). Nursing draws on knowledge and practices that nurses have learnt through experience over time (Emden 1992), as well as using and adapting knowledge and techniques from other established sciences and humanities like anatomy, physiology, sociology and psychology.

Most nurses would also support the concept that nursing care needs to be 'patient-centred', which is identified by Kendall and Lissauer (2003) to be

■ Safe and effective

■ Promote health and well-being

■ Integrated and seamless

■ Informing and empowering

■ Timely and convenient

However, transforming these principles into practice is often difficult. We have already considered how there is still a lack of consensus as to whether nursing should and could be defined, and what nurses should know and do. This is the study of the Philosophy of Nursing and it asks these questions:

■ Is there a coherent set of values or beliefs concerning the nature of nursing?

■ What is nursing? (Vocation, profession, occupation, industry, art, science, craft, discipline.)

■ What could (or should) nursing be? (Ontology, the study of being.)

1.4 So what are values?

Values are complex ideas and they often raise emotions and passion from those who hold 'strong' values about certain things. Values may be espoused; what is expected or assumed to be the 'right' value, in contrast to values-in-use, that is what are actually seen in the behaviour of people as they express their values through action. For example, an espoused value in nursing may be that care should be patient-centred but in reality, if you examine the practices of a busy acute medical ward you may find that tasks such as the drug round are still the central organising feature of the nursing practice rather than the needs of individual patients.

Values can be owned by individuals who may express them as individuals but collective values can also be owned by a group of people, in this case by nursing. Sometimes individual and collective values may come into conflict. Therefore there is a personal challenge to know your own values and to consider your own values in relation to those espoused by nursing.

Beliefs, attitudes and values are related to each other but are also distinct. The power of these constructs, however, often leaves a legacy of ideas from the past and blurs them with the present and future. Beliefs are not necessarily factual but are based on faith, on personal confidence of an idea, a person, an object or a situation. Beliefs may be true some or most of the time but not all of the time. Beliefs may serve as a reliable guide but they do not always involve thinking to the point of certainty. A significant belief within nursing is that care is the essence of nursing. However, not all nurses may share this belief as some nurses may believe that care is only a part of nursing, not its essence. A long-standing public belief is that nurses are angels of mercy. However, in today's nursing that is highly skilled, this spiritual image on its own is not necessarily welcomed. Also there have been significant legal cases which have proved this not to be a universal feature of nurses, such as the 23-year-old nurse Beverly Allit, convicted for murder in 1993 of four children in her care.

Attitudes, however, represent more of a settled behaviour, relatively constant feelings towards a person, an object, an idea or a situation. In relation to nursing, it can be argued that significant attitudes within nursing include compassion, commitment and care to others. However, significant attitudes about nursing could be quite mixed from nursing being seen as an essential backbone service of the National Health Services (NHS) to being a redundant occupation which should modernise.

Values can be changeable, influenced by different situations such as changes in society and experiences through life. When decisions arrive in our lives, turning points make us think and deliberate, we are forced to consider and possibly challenge our values. We normally have values about things that have worth to us. Values colour the way we think about everything in our lives and normally steer our actions. We may have values about what constitutes happiness, health and maturity, about life and death and how we should live in society. However, when they are tested in our lives we may not always behave as we might intend. For example, a person may be positively opposed to euthanasia due to the higher value they have for life. However, if faced with a long-standing painful and inevitable death, it might then seem as a desirable option as the value of reducing suffering may take precedence over the value of life.

Values can define us as persons. 'Values are closely related to meaning – the meaning of life. The inner meaning of an action, an experience or an attitude gives us our values' (Tschudin 1992: 2). In this sense, to seek our values, to find what they really are, we need to question meanings we hold about our actions and experiences, as when the meaning is known the value is known. This questioning can be uncomfortable and uncertain but it can also help us to appreciate our values and assist us with understanding ourselves better and therefore engage with others more knowingly. This is important as we normally live by our values and if we do not know what they are it could give us some complex surprises. Consider your values in Activity 1.3.

ACTIVITY 1.3

Divide a piece of paper into three columns. Head each column up with:

Beliefs   Attitudes   Values

Consider your beliefs, attitudes and values about nursing.
See if you can write these down under the three columns and whether you can identify what influences led you to have these decisions?

Can you consider a time when your values have been challenged and you made a decision to behave in a way that went against your personal values?

In thinking about where your values came from, you probably reflected on how they have been shaped from a variety of internal and external factors, your genetic inheritance, the environments in which you have lived, the influence of people who have been role models, either positive or negative, friends, neighbours and relatives, employment you have experienced, the society in which you were bought up and the society in which you live now. The safest way to engage with our values is to explore issues to make us think about them. This has been a trait promoted by Socrates, who suggested the 'unexamined life is not worth living' (cited in Plato's Apology). This is supportive of being a reflective practitioner in one's personal life as well as in the professional domain (see Chapter 3).

ACTIVITY 1.4

Some people are famous for their values and beliefs. They have clearly stated their values and taken action to live by them. Think of the following people: Mahatma Gandhi, Martin Luther King, Adolph Hitler, Florence Nightingale. Write down what you think their values were and how their values influenced the lives of others.

A personal value system is often akin to a person's morals. It is often guided by 'oughts' and 'shoulds' and is constantly revised through life experiences (see Chapter 5). Importantly, however, the personal values we hold impact on the relationships we have with other people. We can start by trying to identify our own values, first in relation to ourselves and second in relation to nursing.

ACTIVITY 1.5A

Complete the following lines to learn a little about your personal values

The most important aspect of my life is _____
I would reach satisfaction in my life if I could _____
In general, I would say people are _____
People are motivated by _____
All people need _____
The world would be more perfect if _____
Conflicts occur amongst people because _____

Now complete the following lines in Activity 1.5B to see if you can identify the values that guided your decision to train as a nurse.

ACTIVITY 1.5B

I chose nursing because it _____

In my role as a nurse I see myself as _____

Nurses help others because _____

Nurses should interact with clients and patients through _____

I would most like to achieve _____ as a nurse

My greatest disappointment as a nurse would be if I _____

Your transition from student to registered nurse will involve understanding the values of the profession. These may sit comfortably with your own values or you may have tensions with some of them. You will become increasingly aware that becoming a nurse is not simply a matter of learning particular skills, but of adopting forms of behaviour appropriate to a particular context. It is also about coming to know the values of nursing which may influence your thinking and lifestyle. The NMC's Code of Professional Conduct: standards for conduct, performance and ethics (NMC 2004b) is cited as the definitive document that illustrates the espoused shared values of nursing. It cites seven major 'must dos' (see Box 1.2) in the context of accountability of individual nurses and their duty of care to patients and clients. Most countries have their own codes to guide their registered health professionals (see Chapter 5).

BOX 1.2 NMC Code of Professional Conduct: Standards for conduct, performance and ethics (NMC 2004b)

As a registered nurse, midwife or specialist community public health nurse, you are personally accountable for your practice. In caring for patients and clients, you must:

- Respect the patient or client as an individual

- Obtain consent before you give any treatment or care

- Protect confidential information

- Co-operate with others in the team

- Maintain your professional knowledge and competence

- Be trustworthy

- Act to identify and minimise risk to patients

Activity 1.6 invites you to consider the NMC code (NMC 2004b).

ACTIVITY 1.6

Visit the NMC website (www.nmc.org.uk). Check and download the student and the registered nurse version of the professional code. Can you see any potential issues with any of these values in relation to your own? It might be helpful to have a discussion in your tutorial/learning group about this code.

It is interesting how values can change over time so at this point we will turn our attention to the origin of nursing to consider the historical influences of people, society and politics.

1.5 What are the origins of nursing?

The existence of nursing can be traced to the ancient times of the Greeks and Romans. However, some of the earliest accounts of people being organised to care for the sick were in the first century AD, when women called deaconesses visited the sick and needy in their homes (Baly 1994, Hart 2004). Religious orders – often men – dominated this scene as in addition to visiting the sick, they cared for them in special houses attached to monasteries. However, infections could not be contained and so people with what were considered contagious diseases were isolated (e.g. lepers) and wealthy patrons were encouraged to build or 'endow' hospitals and almshouses for the poor, sick, insane, old, feeble or orphans.

In the United Kingdom, several historic hospital foundations were created in this way like St Bartholomew's (1123), St Thomas' (1215) and the Bethlehem Hospital for the mentally ill. Following the dissolution of the monasteries under the Tudors, the first secular laws to ensure that relief was provided at 'parish' level were introduced and five 'Royal' hospitals in London were created from former religious foundations. The staff of these institutions now became employed lay people (usually women) who were recruited from the marketplace and were of variable quality. This 'parish' system, relying on personal and civic responsibility, was common in Protestant countries and worked until people began to move from their parishes to the towns and cities (urbanisation).

The division of labour in illness was influenced by industrialisation, urbanisation and gender. The first factory was invented, designed and opened by Sir Richard Arkwright in the 1770s. It bought a new focus on time, shift working, the breakdown of complex manufacturing to production of items into simple tasks with individuals separated from the whole product like never before, employment of supervisors to watch over the workers and waged employment (Maggs 2002). Urbanisation followed the growth of employment opportunities in factories, which led to cramped unhealthy conditions and a rise in disease, ill health and accidents. Workhouses developed and hospitals were required, which dovetailed with better transportation and the development of scientific, medical knowledge which began to change the status of doctors. Doctors gradually professionalised and this was confirmed with the Medical Act of 1958. The legacy associated with Florence Nightingale and Mrs Bedford Fenwick and the effects of the workhouses and new hospitals were to have significant impact upon United Kingdom nursing in the early twentieth century.

ACTIVITY 1.7

In your local area, find out when the first hospital was built, by whom and why. Is it still operating and if not, why not? Was the first hospital a Royal, Charity, Voluntary, Religious or Military Hospital, a former workhouse or a 'new' hospital built since the introduction of the NHS in 1949?

To help you, find out from the university or your local authority librarian if there is a local archive, historian or history of nursing in your locality.

Nursing in the United Kingdom is still predominantly a female occupation unlike other countries such as Malta. Nursing is 'gendered as it espouses values and systems associated with women, which are constructed rather than biologically determined' (Maggs 2002: 14). As the female population rose, there was a steady stream of volunteers from respectable families to join hospitals as nurses, with the core distinction in hospitals between the women who were the nurses and the men who were the doctors. Before the twentieth century, nursing included not just caring for the sick and the wounded associated with wars, but also doing tasks associated with housekeeping and domestic work. The practice of nurses working under the *direct* supervision of the medical staff developed with the expansion of medical knowledge and the rise of medical control in hospitals and public or primary health care during the nineteenth century (see Hart 2004).

Nightingale, the Protestant Deaconesses and other religious-inspired individuals or groups (like Roman Catholic nuns) expressed their nursing through their 'vocation' and belief in God. They helped to transform the image of nursing through their high standards of practice, their concepts of duty, codes of behaviour and the importance of learning subjects like nutrition, anatomy and physiology, medicine, sanitation, hygiene and communication/comfort skills. Their 'mission' of intelligent, competent practice spread through many parts of Europe and the world. However, the hierarchical, sometimes convent- or military-like nursing environments governed by matrons (Lady Superintendents) from the sixteenth century were questioned in the twentieth century as women's roles expanded, women's liberation was kindling and secularisation was increasing with society becoming less hierarchical itself.

1.6 Florence Nightingale, Mrs Bedford Fenwick and Political action

Florence Nightingale is famous as the 'Lady of the Lamp' from her work in Scutari Hospital during the Crimean War. Together with influential friends, she had a major impact on the development of the organisation of the hospital as an institution (Maggs 2002), the establishment of nursing schools and reforms of the 'Poor Laws'. Her landmark work 'Notes on Nursing' (Nightingale 1970: 8) considered that she used the term *nursing* 'for want of any better' and that the 'very elements of nursing are all but unknown'. This leaves us the legacy of the debates as to what nursing is. Other women who were also very influential in developing nursing include Mary Jane Seacole, Mrs Mackenzie and Elizabeth Davis (see Chapter 2 in Ardern 2002). Some of these women were 'rejected' by Nightingale as they exhibited different values.

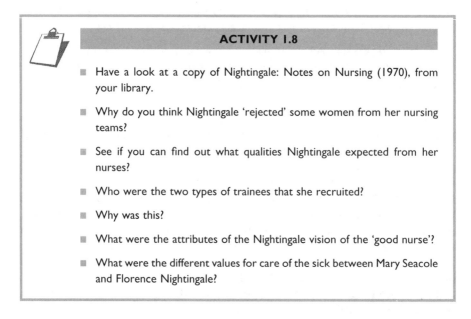

ACTIVITY 1.8

■ Have a look at a copy of Nightingale: Notes on Nursing (1970), from your library.

■ Why do you think Nightingale 'rejected' some women from her nursing teams?

■ See if you can find out what qualities Nightingale expected from her nurses?

■ Who were the two types of trainees that she recruited?

■ Why was this?

■ What were the attributes of the Nightingale vision of the 'good nurse'?

■ What were the different values for care of the sick between Mary Seacole and Florence Nightingale?

Mrs Bedford Fenwick (nee Ethel Gordon Manson) epitomised a secular, professional approach to nursing (Bradshaw 1994). She had been the matron at St Bartholomew's hospital and was one of the main leaders of the movement to 'register' nurses in a way similar to doctors. This required the introduction of a national examination and registration scheme for nurses. Nightingale opposed this development stating that if introduced too early it would lead to low standards and that a national examination could not test the right personal qualities and aptitudes. In contrast, Mrs Bedford Fenwick claimed that registration was a way to lengthen the training, raise the standards and esteem of nursing, protect the 'new' nurses and raise the status of women. Others thought the fees would be too high, that the new standards would mean fewer recruits and that the registrants could take work away from doctors.

To introduce compulsory registration required an Act of Parliament, and so nursing became the subject of political activity and debate. At the same time, Mrs Bedford Fenwick was instrumental in launching several nursing organisations to apply pressure for change: the Matron's Council (1894), the British Nurses Association (1897) and the International Council of Nurses (1899).

Opponents helped to form the College of Nursing (1916), which is now the Royal College of Nursing.

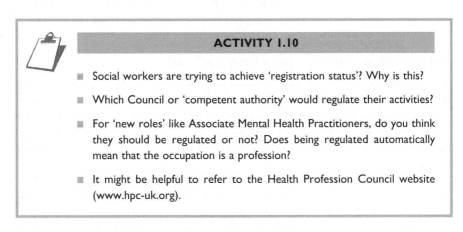

ACTIVITY 1.9

Consider why was it important to form these various associations? Consider how powerful some of them became, and are. Why, at its inception, did the College of Nursing not admit men and have rules to prevent it becoming a Trade Union?

As nursing was wrestling to identify itself as a vocation or a developing profession, the arguments over the control of nursing were in full swing. This was all taking place in the context of the British Empire, the introduction of compulsory education for children, a succession of military conflicts (Boer War, First World War), a demand for large numbers of semi-trained women to care for the casualties of war and the struggle for women's suffrage. Finally in 1919, nurse registration was achieved through an Act of Parliament (Nurses Registration Act 1919), with a General Nursing Council to act as the 'competent authority' to control nursing and ensure public protection. At this time there were special 'Parts' of the Register for those qualified to give general care, and nurse sick children or those with mental diseases. There was a special section for male nurses. These debates concerning the standard of nursing, the 'Parts' of the register and the nature of nurse education have continued over the century and are still as alive today as they were in the early 1900s. The most recent revision of the register took place in 2004 with three parts being now in statute: qualified nurses, midwives and specialist community public health nurses.

Activity 1.10 encourages you to consider other related occupations which are not currently regulated the same way as nursing.

ACTIVITY 1.10

■ Social workers are trying to achieve 'registration status'? Why is this?

■ Which Council or 'competent authority' would regulate their activities?

■ For 'new roles' like Associate Mental Health Practitioners, do you think they should be regulated or not? Does being regulated automatically mean that the occupation is a profession?

■ It might be helpful to refer to the Health Profession Council website (www.hpc-uk.org).

Since 1919, nursing has been a regulated occupation in the United Kingdom but two principles of the increasingly influential European Union (EU) have particular importance for nursing. First, there is the principle of 'freedom of movement' that entitles citizens of one EU country to live and work in another EU country. The second principle follows from this, namely that states should mutually recognise the academic and professional qualifications held by European citizens. In the interests of public safety, occupations like medicine, nursing and midwifery have European Laws that govern their training to ensure a minimum standard across Europe. British nurses played a key role in the 1960s and 1970s in establishing these regulations. The programmes designed to enable general nurses to practise in the discipline are subject to two Sectoral directives relating to the qualifications of 'nurses responsible for general care'. These are Directive 77/453/EEC of 27 June 1977 and Directive 89/595/EEC of 10 October 1989 and are summarised in counsel 1977L0453 dated 31/7/2001. This means that, subject to being up to date and competent in the language and culture, a nurse trained in another EU country would have his/her registration as a general nurse automatically recognised. Since the introduction of the Adult Branch of nursing, the 'general nurse' directive has been applied to adult nursing. Other specialities in nursing are subject to what are called general system directives, therefore do not have automatic mutual recognition of their professional qualification.

Let us focus a little more on the education and training of nurses in the context of thinking about what should nurses know and do.

ACTIVITY 1.11

■ When was training or education for nurses first introduced in your area? Did the student nurses pay for their training or were they paid to train, or was it a combination of the two?

■ To help you, find out from the university or your local authority librarian if there is a local archive, historian or history of nursing in your locality.

1.7 What should nurses know and do?

The current requirements on what nurses should know and do are presented as 'standards' by the NMC (NMC 2004a) in line with the Nursing and Midwifery Order 2001 (Statutory Instrument 2004/254; see Section 1.2.1, and go to the NMC website www.nmc-uk.org). These standards are supported through education programmes approved by the NMC which involve practice and academic studies.

This dual model of practice and study is not new but student nurses originally learnt 'what to do and why' as apprentices rather than as supernumery students, by being taught practical nursing under the supervision of nurse tutors, ward sisters and other nurses. They would also receive instruction and study knowledge from other disciplines, for example medicine, pharmacy, anatomy, physiology and, from the 1960s onwards, also the social sciences. 'Duties of care' and codes of conduct were taught together with ethics and relevant laws and after Nightingale in the early Nineteenth century, techniques of management, hygiene, nutrition, housekeeping and public health. With the advances of science and other disciplines like management and organisational studies, nursing education has been under pressure to apply 'new' knowledge to nursing. However, as Macleod Clark and Hockey (1988: 6) described, nurses were initially 'largely dependent on members of other disciplines, especially the social sciences for the study of their own profession'. Sometimes of course, these disciplines may have been inappropriate for the nursing context. However, the enduring question is whether nursing has its own unique and distinct knowledge base. This study of the types and nature of knowledge used by nurses is epistemology. It is the branch of philosophy concerned with the nature of knowledge, the scope of knowledge and the general source or basis of knowledge(Cameron-Traub 1991).

Carper (1978), a nurse academic, suggests that there are four fundamental patterns, or types, of knowing in nursing, namely

1. Empirics or the science of nursing (e.g. why do pressure sores occur?)

2. Aesthetics or the art of nursing (e.g. how does one reassure a patient, or make someone comfortable using pillows?)

3. Personal knowledge – the knowledge that an individual has about themselves and the way they can use themselves in their nursing practice (knowledge based on experience and self-awareness)

4. Ethics and the moral component – the 'rights', 'wrongs' and uncertainties of decision making (e.g. whether someone should be resuscitated or not).

Gobbi (2005) argues that while nurses may use these types of knowledge, in practice, they often 'cobble' them together to address real, concrete situations in practice. When this happens and nurses bring together knowledge from the sciences, humanities, personal knowledge/experience, ethics, artistry and traditions or ritual to deal with practice issues and client care, they are acting as *bricoleurs*. This term was first used by the anthropologist Claude Lévi-Strauss, who argued that bricoleurs were practical people who used whatever was at hand to deal with the current 'task'. In so doing, they were often imaginative and creative, using knowledge and tools in ways for which they were not designed.

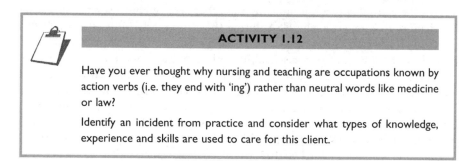

ACTIVITY 1.12

Have you ever thought why nursing and teaching are occupations known by action verbs (i.e. they end with 'ing') rather than neutral words like medicine or law?

Identify an incident from practice and consider what types of knowledge, experience and skills are used to care for this client.

Nursing slowly began its entry into academia in the 1950s but in the United Kingdom it was only with the advent of Project 2000 in 1989 (UKCC 1986) that the link between higher education and training was firmly rooted. Due to their earlier start, North American nurses became the initial nurse theorists who pioneered writing down their theories about nursing and developing conceptual models to guide nurses in their practice. They also invented the phrase, 'nursing process' (Yura and Walsh 1967) to encourage nurses to demonstrate in a logical and systematic approach how they assessed, planned, implemented and evaluated their individualised care for patients and clients (see Chapter 2). It must be remembered that up until this time, nursing had held a traditional oral culture where specific nursing knowledge was passed from one nurse to another in pratice, usually within a hierarchical culture.

At the heart of these nursing theories are the values, beliefs and sources of knowledge that have influenced their development. The range and number (over 50) of nursing theories that have been published is remarkable, reflecting the different conceptual positions of the authors which are often gained from their own educational and practice experience backgrounds. These issues are well presented by Kitson (1993), where the nurse theory protagonists (Abdellah *et al.* 1973, Hall 1977, Henderson 1978, Orem 1980) began a needs-based orientation to practice which was historically situated. Peplau (1952) developed this further through emphasising the explicit importance of the nurse–patient relationship, which caught the imagination of the second group of nurse theorists such as King (1981), Orlando (1961) and Travelbee (1971). They reduced the focus on the physical needs of patients in favour of the therapeutic use of self, establishing a relation based on trust, equality and mutual regard (Kitson 1993). Outcome theories, as described by Meleis (1985) were the next to be developed with Roy (1976), drawing on adaptation theory as the most famous in the United Kingdom. Useful as these theories are for developing distinct knowledge, the models for practice that accompanied them based on the theories were complex and difficult to put into practice, both conceptually and in record keeping. However, a common feature with all these theories is their models offer 'key components of care' that outline particular ways of viewing the person, the causes of the person's problems, the nature of assessing, planning and evaluating care (nursing process), the role of the nurse and the focus of implementing the nursing care to meet the needs of the patient (Aggleton and Chalmers 2000).

The concept of care has a long association with nursing. Nursing and care are usually put together as nursing care. However, what 'care' means and whether care is the central concept in nursing is another area of controversy. The caring curriculum movement in the USA during the 1980s and 1990s (Watson 1989) tried to secure care as the essence of nursing (Watson 1985, Roach 1987) and to reduce the influence of the scientific method of cause and effect, the medical model of diagnosis and cure and to put the person at the heart of health care. Kitson (1993) traces three conceptual transitions of care in nursing which have coherence with nursing theories, starting from caring-as-duty originating from Nightingale; second is seeing care as a therapeutic relationship; and third is caring-as-ethical position. Benner (1989) is of particular note in the last category where the 'expert' practitioner is not 'bounded by rules' but able to 'make independent judgements on each case within the context of where the care is carried out' (Kitson 1993: 41). In a later paper, she suggests that what nurses should do is to have the appropriate skills and knowledge, a commitment to care for others and respect for the other person's wishes, desires and rights (Kitson 1987). It can be argued that it is the importance of valuing all these elements that defines what nurses should know. There is a need for knowledge from the life and social sciences, there is the need for knowledge about nursing theories, there is the need for practical knowledge in the form of competencies, there is the need for personal knowledge of self to facilitate effective therapeutic relationships, and there is the need for ethical knowledge to promote respect for individuals. As each nurse is a person, however much they learn from external knowledge sources, it is the joint influences of the external culture of nursing and its internalisation, motivation and value system that interpret this knowledge for practice. Such is the expectation on nurses today and the importance of professional studies.

In deciding whether nursing has its own body of knowledge, we have to consider whether there is 'special' knowledge that is unique to nursing and not held by others and whether there are skills or competences that nurses hold in common with others. Barr (2002) identifies different types of competences; there are those that are held in common by all care professions, those that distinguish one profession from another (complementary) and those that are necessary to enable the professionals to work effectively with one another (collaborative). All three types are essential for offering unique but collaborative contributions to patient-centred care. It is useful to reflect on these three types and relate them to nursing as well as to other health and social care roles.

A common feature for all health and social care professionals in the twenty-first century is the importance placed on the use of evidence to inform practice (see Chapters 10–12). In this sense, which discipline developed the evidence is not more important than how robust and relevant the evidence is for the patient(s) or client(s) in question to support well-being and effective health outcomes. In this sense, the collaborative model for knowledge generation is taking precedence. This is also reflected in practice where it is more important that the knowledge and skills of an individual practitioner match the needs of the patient rather than the role (see Chapter 12).

ACTIVITY 1.13

List at least four other health or social care professional roles.

Jot down what you think are the common, complementary and collaborative competences and qualities of these roles.

1.8 Conclusion

Nursing is a dynamic concept which shapes and is shaped by the society which it purports to serve. Nursing does not work as an isolated activity but within a complex health and social framework. Nursing has long been involved in debating its definition, its purpose, its role and its status, but its core values and principles are enduring: to care for others with knowledge, respect and skill. This chapter has begun the journey to explore these principles, starting with thoughts on these questions: What is nursing? What are its values and its knowledge base? What are the origins of nursing? These important questions highlight the continuous journey that nursing is undertaking through the centuries. Your journey is just beginning within nursing and as you travel it is hoped that you are guided by the principles of professional studies in nursing.

SELF-EVALUATION

And, finally, your chance to revise what you have learnt from this chapter

1. What is your personal definition of nursing?

2. Write out three other definitions of nursing and explain their similarities and differences.

3. What are values?

4. Where are the values of nursing most clearly stated?

5. Name Carper's four ways of knowing in nursing.

6. How do different types of knowledge support the practice and discipline of nursing?

7. Which two nurses changed the face of nursing in the United Kingdom – what were their differing perspectives on nursing?

8. Which authority is responsible for the standard of proficieny in nursing practice?

References

Abdellah, F.G., Beland, I.L., Martin, A., and Matheney, R.V. (1973) *New Directions in Patient-centred Nursing: Guidelines for Systems of Service, Education and Research.* Macmillan, New York.

Aggleton, P. and Chalmers, H. (2000) Nursing models and nursing practice (Second edition). Macmillan, Basingstoke.

Ardern, P. (2002) *When Matron Ruled.* Hale, London.

American Nurses Association (ANA) (1980) *Nursing: A Social Policy Statement.* ANA, Kansas City.

Baly, M.E. (1994) *Nursing and Social Change.* Routledge, London.

Barr, H. (2002) *A Critical Review of Evaluations of Interprofessional Education.* Centre for Health Sciences and Practice. Occasional Paper 2. LTSN, London.

Benner, P. (1989) *From Novice to Expert: Excellence and Power in Clinical Nursing Practice.* Addison Wesley, London.

Bradshaw, A. (1994) *Lighting the Lamp: The Spiritual Dimension of Nursing Care.* Scutari Press, London.

Cameron-Traub, E. (1991) An evolving discipline. In: Gray, G. and Pratt, R. (eds) *Towards a Discipline of Nursing.* Churchill Livingstone, Melbourne.

Carper, B.A. (1978) Fundamental patterns of knowing in nursing. *Advances in Nursing Science* 1: 13–23.

Department of Health (DOH) (1999a) *The New NHS: Modern and Dependable*. HMSO, London.

Department of Health (DOH) (1999b) *Making a Difference*. HMSO, London.

Department of Health (DOH) (2004a) *The Knowledge and Skills Framework*. HMSO, London.

Department of Health (DOH) (2004b) *Agenda for Change*. HMSO, London.

Emden, C. (1992) Ways of knowing in nursing. In: Gray, G. and Pratt, R. (eds) *Towards a Discipline of Nursing*. Churchill Livingstone, Melbourne.

Gobbi, M. (2005) Nursing practice as bricoleur activity: A concept explored. *Nursing Inquiry* 12(2): 117–125.

Hall, B. (1977) The effect of interpersonal attraction on the therapeutic relationship; a review and suggestion for further study. *Journal of Psychiatric Nursing* 15(9): 18–23.

Hart, C. (2004) *Nurses and Politics: The Impact of Power and Practice*. Palgrave Macmillan, Basingstoke.

Henderson, V.A. (1978) *Principles and Practice of Nursing*. Macmillan, USA.

Henderson, V.A. (1991) *The Nature of Nursing: Reflections After 25 Years*. National League for Nursing, New York.

International Council of Nurses (ICN) (1998) *ICN on Regulation: Towards 21st Century Models*. ICN, Geneva.

International Council of Nurses (ICN) (2003) ICN framework of competences for the generalist nurse. ICN, Geneva.

International Labour Conference (63rd: 1977: Geneva). Employment and conditions of work and life of nursing personnel/sixth item on the agenda [of the] International Labour Conference, 63rd session, 1977. Geneva: ILO, 1977.

Kendall, L. and Lissauer, R. (2003) *The Future Health Care Worker*. Institute of PPR, London.

King, I.M. (1981) *A Theory for Nursing: Systems, Concepts, Process*. John Wiley, New York.

Kitson, A.L. (1987) A comparative analysis of lay caring and professional (nursing) caring relationships. *International Journal of Nursing Studies* 24(2): 155–165.

Kitson, A.L. (1993) *Nursing: Art and Science*. Chapman and Hall, London.

Macleod Clark, J. and Hockey, E. (1988) *Research for Nursing: A Guide for the Enquiring Nurse* (Education for care). Scutari Press, London.

Maggs, C. (2002) Milestones in British nursing. In: Daly, J., Speedy, S., and Jackson, D. (eds) *Contexts of Nursing: An Introduction*. Blackwell Publishing, London.

Meleis, A. (1985) *Theoretical Nursing: Development and Progress*. J.B. Lippincott, Philadelphia.

Nightingale, F. (1970) *Notes on Nursing: What It Is and What It Is Not*. Dover Publications, Dover.

Nursing and Midwifery Council (NMC) (2004a) *Standards of Proficiency for Pre-registration Nursing Education*. NMC, London.

Nursing and Midwifery Council (NMC) (2004b) *The NMC Code of Professional Conduct: Standards for Conduct, Performance and Ethics*. NMC, London.

Orem, D. (1980) *Nursing: Concepts of Practice*. McGraw-Hill, New York.

Orlando, I. (1961) *The Dynamic Nurse-Patient Relationship*. G.P. Putman and Sons, New York.

Paterson, J.G. and Zderad, L.T. (1976) *Humanistic Nursing*. Wiley, New York.

Peplau, H. (1952) *Interpersonal Relations in Nursing*. G.P. Putman and Sons, New York.

Quinn, D. and Russell, S. (1993) *Nursing the European Dimension*. Scutari Press, London.

Roach, S. (1987) *The Human Act of Caring*. Canadian Hospital Association, Ottawa.

Rolfe, G. (2000) *Research, Truth, Authority*. Macmillan Press, Basingstoke.

Roy, C. (1976) *Introduction to Nursing: An Adaptation Model*. Prentice-Hall, Englewood Cliffs.

Royal College of Nursing (2003) *Defining Nursing*. RCN, London.

Stokes, M. (1997) *Plato's Apology*. Aris and Phillips, London.

Travelbee, J. (1971) *Interpersonal Aspects of Nursing*. FA Davis, Philadelphia.

Tschudin, V. (1992) *Values*. Balliere Tindall, London.

United Kingdom Central Council for Nursing, Midwifery and Health Visiting (1986) *Project 2000: A New Preparation for Practice*. UKCC, London.

Wanless, D. (2002) *Securing Our Future Health: Taking a Long Term View*. Report to HM Treasury. London.

Watson, J. (1985) *Nursing: The Philosophy and Science of Caring*. Associated University Press, Bolder Colorado.

Watson, J. (1989) A new paradigm of curriculum development. In: Bevis, E. and Watson, J. (eds) *Toward a Caring Curriculum: A New Pedagogy for Nursing*. National League for Nursing, New York.

Whittington, D. and Boore, J. (1988) Competence in nursing. In: Ellis, R. (ed.) *Professional Competence and Quality Assurance in the Caring Professions*. Chapman and Hall, London.

Yura, H. and Walsh, M. (1967) *The Nursing Process*. Appleton-Century-Crofts, Norwalk.

@ Useful websites

www.who   World Health Organisation.

http://www.statistics.gov.uk   United Kingdom Government Office of National Statistics.

www.ilo.org   International Labour Organisation.

www.rcn.org.uk   Royal College of Nursing.

www.nmc-uk.org   Nursing and Midwifery Council.

www.hpc-uk.org   Health Professions Council (13 professions on registers).

www.pcnweb.org   Standing Committee of Nurses in the European Union.

http://www.icn.ch/mailorderRegulation.pdf   International Council of Nurses (Regulations).

http://www.icn.ch/icncode.pdf   International Council of Nurses (Codes).

@ Websites for European education tuning project

http://europa.eu.int/comm/education/policies/educ/tuning/tuning_en.html

http://www.relint.deusto.es/TuningProject/index.htm

📖 Suggested reading

Baly, M.E. (1994) *Nursing and Social Change*. Routledge, London.
A seminal text which offers you greater understanding of the interface between social change and nursing.

Hart, C. (2004) *Nurses and Politics: The Impact of Power and Practice*. Palgrave Macmillan, Basingstoke.
A contemporary text which offers insight into the connection between nursing and politics and deeper appreciation of how change is influenced.

Hogston, R. and Simpson, P. (eds) (2002) *Foundations Studies in Nursing*. Palgrave Macmillan, Basingstoke.
This book offers student nurses a sound basis for understanding clinical practice.

Robinson, J. (2005) *Mary Seacole*. Constable & Robinson, London.
This book offers an account on the life and work of Mary Seacole. It clarifies her values and their influence on her ways of practising nursing, which you can compare to that of Nightingale.

Nursing Theory and Models for Practice

2

Paula Libberton

CONTENTS

- Nursing theory
- Nursing models
- The nursing process
- The medical model
- Roper, Logan and Tierney's activities of living model for nursing
- Roy's adaptation model of nursing

LEARNING OUTCOMES

This chapter should enable you to

- Examine nursing theory
- Discuss nursing models
- Explore the nursing process
- Discuss the medical model of care
- Consider some models of nursing

2.1 Introduction

The aim of this chapter is to set out the relationship between theory and models to allow us to appreciate their contribution to promoting nursing practice. Much has been written about nursing theory and in particular about nursing models, with numerous books emerging in the 1980s. However, it appears that the popularity of nursing theory and its models has diminished over recent years with the emphasis now being placed on interprofessional working and learning. However, it could be argued that nursing practice is inevitably informed by nursing theory. Therefore, it is important that nursing theory is studied to provide us with a better understanding of our everyday practice. First, nursing theory will be considered, then nursing models, followed by a discussion of the nursing process. This is complimented by a brief look at the medical model before considering two examples of nursing models that are currently popular in the United Kingdom. A list of some of the other published nursing models is included to offer direction for further exploration of this vast subject. The chapter ends with a brief exploration of the application of nursing models to current nursing practice.

2.2 What is nursing theory?

'Nursing theory' is really an umbrella term for all of the insights derived from nursing research (Greenwood 2002). This includes conceptual research which goes on in the researcher's head and is responsible for the construction of nursing models, as well as empirical research which is tested out in the real world to inform evidence-based practice. (Evidence-based practice is explored in Chapters 10 and 11.) Theory helps us to make sense of what we observe and perceive by suggesting relationships between concepts which allow us to predict likely future events. It has been described as a map which highlights those parts that are important for the purpose (Stevens Barnum 1998), allowing a person to learn what they need to think about (Visintainer 1986). Greenwood (2002) suggests that theory is a net of concepts constructed to make a person's experiences meaningful and manageable. The knots represent concepts and the strings represent the relationship between these concepts. The relationships between these concepts are termed 'propositions'. It is the completeness and accuracy of the net that reflects the extent to which the person is able to manage and find meaning in the experience. Simply, theory is a logically interconnected set of propositions used to describe, explain and predict the real world (Riehl and Roy 1980). (See Rose and Marks-Maran 1997: 149 for further discussion of definitions of theory in nursing.)

According to Dickoff *et al.* (1968), theory can be divided into four levels: factor-isolating, factor-relating, situation-isolating and situation-producing. The first level is concerned with the identification of factors and variables. The second level tries to offer an explanation of the situation by identifying possible relationships between factors. The third level is about predicting what may happen if factors are varied or manipulated (cause and effect). The fourth level is considered the most sophisticated as it presupposes the existence of theory in the three previous levels. This fourth level of theory has a clear purpose with prescribed actions to achieve a desired goal. Walker and Avant (1996) suggest that these

Table 2.1 Levels of theory, corresponding description and practice example

Level 1 **Description**	Factor-isolating	Patient has a wound that is hot, red, swollen and painful.
Level 2 **Explanation**	Factor-relating	The hotness, redness and swelling may be inflammation and related to an infection.
Level 3 **Prediction**	Situation-relating	Cleaning the wound may reduce the infection and associated pain.
Level 4 **Prescription**	Situation-producing	A clean wound avoids infection.

Source: Adapted from Dickoff et al. (1968) and Walker and Avant (1996).

four levels of theory can be described using the following key words: description, explanation, prediction and prescription. Table (2.1) shows the link between Dickoff et al.'s four levels of theory (1968) and their corresponding description by Walker and Avant (1996), with examples of how they relate to practice.

It has been suggested that there are four levels of theory development in nursing (Walker and Avant 1996). These are metatheory, grand theory, middle-range theory and practice theory. Metatheory is the process of developing theory. In nursing, it is concerned with philosophical methodological aspects of theory building (the epistemology). Grand theory defines nursing from a global perspective and is what most nurses refer to as nursing models or conceptual frameworks (Fawcett 1984). Different ideas of theorists about the goals and structure of nursing practice are articulated through nursing models (Green-wood 2002). Four areas of conceptual commonality have been identified as existing in all of nursing's grand theories (Fawcett 1984). These are termed 'meta-paradigms' and include person, environment, health and nursing (these are discussed further under 'What are nursing models?'). Grand theories are extremely difficult, if not impossible, to test due to their generality (Fawcett and Downs 1986). Middle-range theory, on the other hand, is more testable due to it containing a limited number of variables, although it may still contain elements of a grand theory. Practice theory is the last level of theory development. It identifies a desired goal and what action is required to achieve that goal (Greenwood 2002). It can be compared to Dickoff et al.'s (1968) last level of theory, which is situation-producing theory. Figure (2.1) provides a summary of Walker and Avant (1996) levels of theory development.

It is important to remember that theories can be challenged and changed. We are learning new things every day which challenge our practice and often lead to changes. A classic example stems from the enlightenment period when we once believed that the sun revolved around the earth. However, now we know that the earth, along with several other planets, revolves around the sun. This was, thanks to Copernicus (1473–1543), challenging what we thought we knew (see Copernicus 1995 for a full explanation). Unfortunately, at that time it was not acceptable to express different views and as a result, Copernicus was excommunicated for making his ideas public. An example related to nursing is the earlier thought that rubbing the skin was the best way to prevent pressure

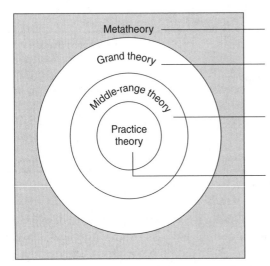

Figure 2.1 Levels of theory development.
Source: Adapted from Walker and Avant (1996).

sores. Now we know from our current understanding of the circulation of the blood that this practice is potentially harmful. This has only arisen by challenging the theory about pressure sore development that was generated some years ago. We need to continue challenging what we think we know in order to ensure that our practice is based on the best available evidence. This may mean thinking outside the box in the same way that Copernicus did but with the knowledge that our challenges will be welcomed and not result in excommunication (Evidence-based practice is discussed further in Chapters 10 and 11).

ACTIVITY 2.1

Can you think of any more examples of theories that have been challenged and subsequently modified? You may remember hearing about examples through the media, reading books and journals or from practice colleagues. What was the original rationale for the theory and what is the new rationale?

(Walsh [1989] offers a range of examples of ritualistic practice [i.e. practice without an evidence base] which has taken place over the years).

2.3 What are nursing models?

So far nursing theory has been discussed with the suggestion that nursing models are grand theories or global theories of nursing. However, there is an argument which suggests that nursing models and nursing theories are at best one and the same (Meleis 1991). According to Fawcett (1995), nursing models are different to nursing theories in that they are rarely testable as a result of their abstract nature. Whereas nursing theories should be able to describe, explain, predict or prescribe phenomena which make it easier to test them for their validity and appropriateness (Walker and Avant 1996). It has been suggested that nursing models may act as the starting point for the development of nursing theory (Aggleton and Chambers 2000), as a model is a set of concepts constructed to guide practice, generate new ideas and differentiate nursing from other professions (Chinn and Jacobs 1983). These arguments serve to demonstrate the difficulty in understanding the relationship between theories and models of nursing. What is clear is that nursing theory and nursing models cannot exist without each other and that each nursing model or theory is built around four basic concepts: person, environment, health and nursing. These concepts are generally considered to be central to the discipline of nursing (Leddy and Pepper 1998). Box 2.1 offers a summary of these concepts.

BOX 2.1 Four concepts of nursing

Person (patient/client)
Environment (society)
Health (or illness)
Nursing (goals, roles, functions)

Source: Adapted from Fawcett (1984).

Although these four concepts can be found in models of nursing, there is wide variation in the amount of emphasis placed on each concept and the theory which might explain the relationship between the concepts (Leddy and Pepper 1998). For example, Roy (1984) views the person as a biopsychosocial being forming a unified system that seeks equilibrium while Parse (1981) defines the person as a patterned, open being, more than and different to the sum of its parts. The environment on the other hand is described by Peplau (1952) in terms of the therapeutic relationship between the nurse and patient whereas Orem (1995) considers the environment in relation to external forces. Health is defined by King (1981) as a dynamic state of well-being while Roper *et al.* (1980) consider health in terms of independence in activities of daily living. Finally, nursing is described by Roy (1984) as the manipulation of stimuli in order to foster successful coping whereas Parse (1981) views nursing as an interactional process that facilitates the becoming of the participants. These brief descriptions of the four concepts as defined by a variety of theorists offer an insight into the multitude of views that people can have about the same thing.

ACTIVITY 2.2

How would you define these four concepts: person, environment, health and nursing?

Models are not peculiar to nursing. We are all familiar with models for different things, for example, a model of a house or a car. These are physical represent-ations which do not necessarily contain all the component parts of the actual house or car but provide a good framework. A nursing model represents reality in a similar way but from the viewpoint of the person creating the model. The model does not exist in the physical world but is an abstract conceptualisation of the way in which nursing happens based on theories. A model of nursing does not have to be formally published by a theorist but can exist informally in all of us. We all have our own concepts and ideas about nursing resulting in a theory or model of nursing. The difficulty with each of us basing our practice on our own model of nursing is that we all have different values and beliefs that we may assume everyone else shares. This is not necessarily useful if we are working as part of a team as it can interfere with the success of the team achieving a desired goal. Formal nursing models have explicit values, beliefs and ways of working, which provides the team with a common framework around which to structure their care.

Beliefs and values play a significant role in nursing (see Chapter 1) as they influence the way in which we undertake nursing practice. As individuals, we all have different beliefs and values which influence the way in which we behave. The beliefs and values that we hold as nurses about people, the environment, health and nursing are important to the way that we practice. Our beliefs and values about these concepts make up what is termed our 'philosophy of care'. We each have our own philosophy of care which influences our practice. It is useful to explore our beliefs and values around nursing so that we are familiar with the philosophy that underpins our practice. As nurses generally work as part of a team with a shared goal, it is logical to assume that the team should share a common philosophy of care. This philosophy of care usually underpins the nursing model that the team has chosen or created (see Johns 1994). Those theorists that have created models of nursing start by exploring and stating their philosophy of care. It is expected that each clinical setting will have a stated philosophy of care which is available to staff, patients/clients and visitors so that they know what the values and beliefs are that underpin the nursing care provided in that particular clinical setting.

ACTIVITY 2.3

Next time you are in a practice setting, find out whether there is a philosophy of care for that setting. Is it displayed for staff, patients/clients and visitors to see? Do you think that practice is based on the stated philosophy of care? What is the evidence for this?

Nursing models can be categorised into three groups based on the major theoret-ical conceptual classification with which the model seems most consistent (Leddy and Pepper 1998). These groups are systems; stress and adaptation; and caring or growth and development. Box 2.2 provides examples of models which fit into these categories. Models based on systems theory consider the changes which result from interactions between all the factors in a situation. King's model (1981), for example, focuses on the interactions of individuals in groups and the influence this behaviour has on the social system. King (1981) sees the purpose of nursing as helping people attain, maintain or restore health. In contrast to systems theory, stress and adaptation theories view change in terms of cause and effect; therefore, a person must adjust to environmental changes to avoid disturbing a balanced existence. Roy's model (1984), for example, suggests that nurses need knowledge of how to help individuals reduce stress and improve their coping strategies in order to adapt to environmental stressors. Models which use caring theory as a framework include Peplau's model (1952), which implies that nurses need to be able to assess an individual's psychosocial needs before they can help them to move forward. The purpose of the model is to foster personality development and key to this process is the interpersonal relationship between the nurse and patient. Box 2.2 not only demonstrates the classification of nursing models according to Leddy and Pepper (1998) but also provides a list of useful references to enable you to explore some of the nursing models in detail.

BOX 2.2 Classification of nursing models

Systems

King, I. (1981) *A Theory for Nursing: Systems, Concepts, Process*. Wiley, New York.

Neuman, B. (1995) *The Neuman Systems Model*. (Third edition) Appleton and Lange, Connecticut.

Stress and adaptation

Roy, C. (1984) *Introduction to Nursing: An Adaptation Model*. Prentice-Hall, New Jersey.

Caring or growth and development

Orem, D. (1995) *Nursing: Concepts of Practice*. Mosby, St Louis.

Parse, R. (1981) *Man-Living-Health: A Theory of Nursing*. Wiley, New York.

Peplau, H. (1952) *Interpersonal relations in Nursing*. Putnam's Sons, New York.

Source: Leddy and Pepper (1998).

ACTIVITY 2.4

Which nursing models have you come across in practice? What is your understanding of the part that they play in providing nursing care?

Essentially, nursing models are systematically constructed frameworks which have been developed in an attempt to provide guidance on the planning and delivery of nursing care (Riehl and Roy 1980). They have scientific foundations which have evolved from nursing observation, from other fields of enquiry or a combination of the two (Fawcett 1995). Nursing models are guides for nursing practice which suggest ways of nursing and caring for people (Walsh 1998). They also define the values with which nurses should work (Aggleton and Chambers 2000). Perhaps most significantly, nursing models distinguish nursing in its own right by providing the external logic to nursing. Nursing models guide nurses in decision-making and enable nurses to work collaboratively as a team with the same aims based on similar beliefs. However, in order for nursing models to be effective, a systematic process is required to deliver care in an ordered and logical manner. The nursing process is the tool of choice.

2.4 What is the nursing process?

The nursing process is in essence a problem-solving framework (Yura and Walsh 1967). It consists of a series of steps which are not particular to nursing. It is a process that is undertaken as many times as required in response to the changing needs of the patient/client. The nursing process can be viewed as a vehicle by which the components of a nursing model are delivered (Pearson *et al.* 2005). The nursing process originated in the United States as a tool for teaching students about holistic care (Walsh 1998). It was introduced to the United Kingdom in the late 1970s as an effective and systematic way of delivering individualised care. The nursing process is a way of thinking about the problems that patients/clients present. It consists of four stages: assessment, planning, implementation and evaluation. More recently, a fifth stage has been introduced between assessment and planning – nursing diagnosis (Christenson and Kenney 1990, 1995). This stage requires the nurse to make a definitive statement about the patient/client's nursing needs. It differs from medical diagnosis in that it emphasises the whole person and not just the disease or illness. See Figure 2.2.

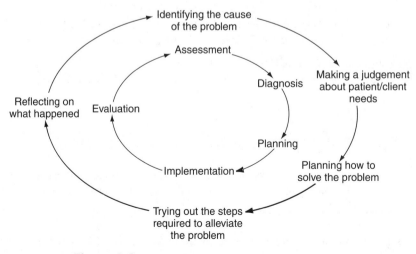

Figure 2.2 The nursing process and problem-solving cycle.

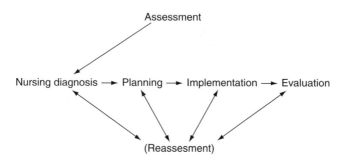

Figure 2.3 The nursing process and reassessment.

The nursing process appears straightforward with the suggestion that there are discrete phases to move through in a particular order. Assessment is always at the start of the process. This informs the nursing diagnosis, planning, implementation and evaluation phases. However, reassessment at any stage of the process can lead to immediate changes in any of these four phases. Assessment is continuous and ongoing and should not be confused with evaluation, which measures outcomes. Assessment and reassessment are about collecting and analysing data to inform nursing care. Therefore it is important to be aware that the nursing process may not follow a set of steps in a linear fashion but may be complicated by the ever changing needs of the patient/client. This is depicted in Figure 2.3.

The nursing process alone is a rather empty approach to care as it encourages nurses to assess but does not tell them what to look for (Aggleton and Chambers 2000). It expects a nursing diagnosis but does not provide a list of diagnoses. It promotes planning but does not provide a template for care planning. It mentions interventions but does not state which interventions to use in which circumstances. Finally, it states that an evaluation should be carried out but it does not offer a discussion of the standards against which this is to be undertaken. In order to use the nursing process effectively, it is necessary to understand and apply appropriate concepts and theories from nursing as well as related disciplines such as the social sciences and life sciences (Paul and Reeves 1995). It is this knowledge which provides the rationale for decision-making, interpersonal relationships and actions in nursing. Together, knowledge of nursing theory, models, the nursing process and related health and social sciences create a framework for providing effective nursing care.

Figure 2.4 offers a diagrammatic representation of the concepts and theories that have been discussed so far within this chapter with the aim of demonstrating how they all link together. This is followed by a brief overview of the medical model before two popular nursing models are discussed.

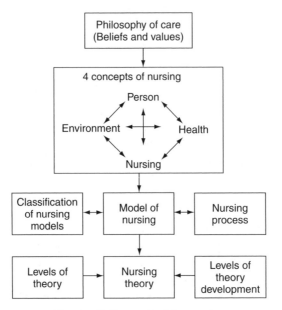

Figure 2.4 How it all fits together.

2.5 The medical model

The medical model of care is familiar to most nurses as it has formed the basis of both medical and nurse training for a number of years. The model purports that a person is a complex set of anatomical parts and physiological systems (Aggleton and Chambers 2000). It places emphasis on the structure and function of the body rather than on the uniqueness and integrity of the individual (Thibodeau 1983). It encourages a disease-orientated approach to care, which focuses on 'putting things right'. Physical and psychological health problems are attributed to a malfunction within the anatomical, physiological or biochemical systems of the body. Therefore, illnesses such as schizophrenia are viewed as resulting from a chemical imbalance which can be corrected by the use of medication. Similarly, other conditions are treated by removing or modifying some anatomical part. This can be seen in the case of cancer, where the diseased tissue or organ is removed in a bid to free the person from disease.

The medical model approach to care is now considered to be inadequate by many nurses and increasing numbers of doctors. This model does not make any allowances for individual needs and therefore only works well with routine and traditional physical care (Downer 2002). It is no longer viewed as an accept-able system of beliefs to understand all health-related needs (Aggleton and Chambers 2000). More importantly, it does not fulfil patients' clients' expect-ations of health care provision. Patients/clients are increasingly encouraged to take responsibility for their health, which means that they are often the experts about their condition and circumstances. Therefore the power that Capra (1982) suggests that the medical model offers doctors can result in a devaluing of know-ledge held by both patients/clients and nurses who are often better placed to make certain decisions. Ideally, care decisions should be made in collaboration with the patient/client, nurse and doctor, with neither striving for power but agreeing on a common goal. Unlike the medical model, most nursing models are based on the assumption that the mind and body are inseparable and that what happens to one part of the body affects the person as a whole entity. It is therefore acknowledged that individuals need holistic care and that we should no longer be treating 'the appendix in bed two', instead we should be caring for 'Mrs X who happens to have an appendicitis'.

ACTIVITY 2.5

What are your views on the medical model? Can you identify the advantages and disadvantages of using this model from a (1) nursing perspective; (2) medical perspective; and (3) patient/client perspective?

2.6 Roper, Logan and Tierney's activities of living model for nursing

It has been suggested that nursing models positively influence practice and therefore should be used in providing care for patients/clients. However, there are many models from which to choose. The model that is used should provide the best approach for the patients'/clients' needs and reflect the clinical area or team philosophy (Walsh 1998). The model that is presented here is intended to provide you with a flavour of what a nursing model is about as so far nursing models have been discussed in general terms.

This model was developed in 1980 from the findings of research undertaken by Nancy Roper in 1976 on the clinical experiences of student nurses. She was particularly interested in developing an idea about nursing that would help students look beyond the medical labels attached to patients/clients to encourage them to view the person holistically. This was the first model of nursing to be developed by British nurses. It is widely used in the United Kingdom particularly in adult nursing. The model is appreciated for its clarity, as most practitioners are able to refer to the original text rather than relying on secondary sources, which often happens when studying more complex American models (Pearson *et al.* 2005).

The model defines the four concepts of nursing as discussed under the heading 'what are nursing models?' people, environment, health and nursing. People are viewed as individuals who are engaged in activities (human needs) that enable them to live and grow throughout a lifespan (which is affected by influencing factors). The environment is considered in terms of where the patient/client is located and the resources that are available to the nurse, which will together influence care planning. Health is defined by independence in activities of living. Interventions by the nurse and patient/client are about supporting independence in these activities by seeking, preventing and comforting. Therefore, nursing is about caring through comforting, seeking and preventing activities as an independent practitioner but where appropriate being dependent or interdependent on a range of other health and social care professionals.

The model is based on Henderson's model of nursing (1966), which defines nursing as helping people with 14 universal human needs. Roper *et al.* (1980) developed a model which focuses on 12 activities which people engage in to live. The starting point for this model is Maslow's hierarchy of human needs (1954), which suggests that unless basic needs are met, such as the need for food and water, people cannot go on to express themselves intellectually or creatively and become self-actualised beings. The activities of daily living can be seen in Box 2.3. They describe relatively distinct types of human behaviour related to meeting a particular need. Some have a biological basis such as eating and drinking whereas others are more socially and culturally determined such as personal dressing and cleansing.

BOX 2.3 The 12 activities of daily living

1. Maintaining a safe environment

2. Communicating

3. Breathing

4. Eating and drinking

5. Eliminating

6. Personal cleansing and dressing

7. Controlling body temperature

8. Mobilising

9. Working and playing

10. Expressing sexuality

11. Sleeping

12. Dying

Source: Roper *et al.* (1980).

These activities of daily living are set against an independence–dependence continuum related to lifespan. It is recognised that people involve themselves in activities of living in different ways depending on the stage in their life. The continuum can be used to plot the activities of daily living and work out where on the independence–dependence continuum the person is trying to return. The activities of living are considered to be influenced by five factors: biological, psychological, sociocultural, environmental and politico-economic. In addition to these factors, there are three types of activities which are closely related to the 12 activities of living. These are preventing, comforting and seeking activities. Nurses and patients/clients may act in preventing certain situations from arising as well as seeking activities to minimise dependence and promote independence. Nurses will also comfort patients/clients and those associated with them.

The model has been refined and developed over time. It has moved away from a disease-based approach to care which originated from the medical model. Nursing has been redefined to emphasise its role in preventing, alleviating and coping with problems associated with activities of daily living. It also gives more consideration to the cultural, environmental, political and economic factors affecting health. However, although this model remains popular in Britain, it has been criticised for focusing on the physical aspects of care even though it does identify broader influencing factors. It has been suggested that the reductionist approach taken by the model is not in keeping with the concept of holism (Jasper 2002). Indeed, some nurses may consider the concept of nursing depicted within this model to be short-sighted as it does not cover many aspects of the work carried out by nurses who find themselves outside a hospital-based adult setting. Nonetheless, the model was developed with the intention that it could be used in a variety of different clinical areas. (See Fraser [1996] for an account of the different practice areas where this model has been shown to be effective.)

ACTIVITY 2.6

The branch of nursing that you are studying will determine whether you come across Roper, Logan and Tierney's activities of living model for nursing in practice. However, it would be useful for you to further explore this model to see how a model can be used in practice. Think of a patient/client that you have nursed and consider how this model may have influenced care positively or negatively.

Roper, N., Logan, W., Tierney, A., and Holland, K. (2004) *Applying the Roper-Logan-Tierney Model in Practice: Elements of Nursing*. Churchill Livingstone, London.

2.7 Roy's adaptation model of nursing

This model of nursing was developed in the 1960s by Callista Roy in the United States and put into use in 1970. It has since become popular in the United Kingdom, particularly in the field of mental health nursing (Downer 2002) where Roper, Logan and Tierney's model was seen to be lacking because of its emphasis on physical care (Murphy *et al.* 2000). The model is influenced by Roy's knowledge of systems theory (von Bertalanffy 1968) and adaptation theory (Helson 1964). Roy developed the idea that people should be viewed as a whole system that responds or adapts to changes or stimuli. These stimuli can be found within the person or in the surrounding environment. Pearson *et al.* (2005) suggest that Roy's rational for using this model is that it enhances patient/client-centred care and supports the concept of accountability for nursing as a scientific discipline. Although the model has not been scientifically proven, Roy maintains that the beliefs upon which the model is based are generally accepted as being true. The model is usually known as Roy's adaptation model because of the strong emphasis on adaptation (Aggleton and Chambers 2000).

According to Pearson *et al.* (2005), Roy views people as individuals who are made up of a number of interrelated systems which together make them whole. The three main systems are biological, psychological and social systems. These systems are in constant interaction with each other and the environment. They should not be looked at as parts that make up the person. Instead, we should focus on the behaviours and responses of the individual to ill health within the systems. The idea is that each system is striving for stability within itself, in relation to other systems and the broader environment. It is recognised that there is no single perfect state of homeostasis which is applicable to everyone as we are all individuals. Therefore it is vital that nurses work with the individuality of each person. In order to maintain this balance people adapt to changes or stimuli. These stimuli have been categorised into three groups: (1) focal – things that have an immediate effect such as the sudden onset of a serious illness; (2) contextual – things within the environment which may result in a negative response to the focal stimulus, for example social isolation and financial difficulties; and (3) residual – beliefs and attitudes resulting from past experiences which may affect the current response, for example 'I should be grateful that I am still alive therefore I will not bother the nurses with my fears of being so unwell'.

Rambo (1984) explains that people react to situations within what Roy terms an individual 'adaptation zone'. As long as the stimuli affecting that person fall within their adaptation zone, that person's integrity will be maintained. This is seen as an adaptive or positive response. If the stimuli are overwhelming, the adaptations made in response may not be sufficient to maintain homeostasis. This is considered to be a maladaptive or negative response. Each person's adaptation zone is of a different size. Therefore, one person may consider the loss of a job to be an opportunity to do something different in life – a positive adaptation response. Another person may think it is the end of the world and experience a debilitating depressive episode – a negative adaptation response. In order to maintain integrity, it is suggested that people have certain needs, which Roy divides into four modes: (1) physiological – concerned with the structure and function of the body; (2) self-concept – associated with the way we perceive ourselves; (3) role function – related to our role and society's expectations of us and (4) interdependence – involved with the balance between independence and dependency on others. Roy sees health and illness on a continuum, with movement along this continuum a normal part of life. A person becomes unwell when the responses they make fall outside the adaptation zone either because they do not have sufficient energy or the stimuli are overwhelming. Therefore, health is maintained as a result of enough energy and the ability to make positive adaptation responses which fall within the person's adaptation zone. The terminology used by Roy is quite different to that with which most people are familiar. Therefore, you may find it necessary to read this section more than once before you have a true grasp of the model. In addition, you will need to consult the book by Andrews and Roy (1997) for an in-depth discussion of the model before you consider using it in practice.

ACTIVITY 2.7

Roy emphasises adaptation as the key to her model. Next time you are in practice, choose a patient/client and see if you can identify whether the person's response to stimuli (changes) is adaptive or maladaptive. You could try this activity on yourself at a time when you feel particularly stressed or observe one of your colleagues in a similar situation.

2.8 Models of nursing

There are many models of nursing to choose from depending on your patient/client group and setting. It is not possible to discuss all of the models in this chapter so instead a list of some of the published models and associated literature is provided. These are not the original texts but have been selected because they offer a modern interpretation of the model to make it more appropriate to contemporary practices.

Neuman's systems model of nursing
Neuman, B. and Fawcett, J. (2001) *The Neuman Systems Model.* Prentice Hall, New Jersey.

Orem's self-care model of nursing
Orem, D. (1995) *Nursing: Concepts of Practice.* Mosby, St Louis.

Peplau's development model of nursing
Simpson, H. (1991) *Peplau's Model in Action.* Macmillan, Basingstoke.

Riehl's interaction model of nursing
Kershaw, B. and Price, B. (1993) *The Riehl Interaction Model in Action.* Palgrave Macmillan, Basingstoke.

ACTIVITY 2.8

To increase your understanding of models of nursing and to help you decide which model is best for your patients/clients, it is important to have explored more than one published model. Consider reading about one of the models in the list provided or select another model that has caught your attention. Prepare a small presentation that you can deliver to your colleagues to increase all of your awareness of the model.

2.9 The application of nursing models to current practice

It is acknowledged that there is little good quality evidence to support the use of nursing models as this area has not been the focus of much research activity (Fraser 1996). However, there are benefits of using a nursing model. It is suggested that discussing beliefs and values about nursing in itself leads to increased commitment and motivation, resulting in nurses feeling that they are part of a team. The introduction and use of a nursing model may also lead to less conflict, as well as encouraging continuity and consistency of care, as nurses are working to the same beliefs and values. The use of a model can also assist in identifying deficiencies in care as it offers a framework against which to set standards which can be easily evaluated.

Models usually require that specific documentation is completed to chart the progress of the patient/client. This is of particular importance as it forces nurses to be accountable for the care that they provide. There is now an expectation that nurses will document their decision-making, which did not happen prior to the 1970s when nursing models had not been formally developed. It is helpful if nurses working with a particular model share the beliefs and values of that model. However, even if they do not they should be able to work according to the model as it will lead the care that they are providing as part of a team. It is not necessary for nurses to use a published nursing model, instead it may be more appropriate for a model to be created to meet the needs of the client group in a particular care setting.

It may be appropriate to analyse and evaluate a number of nursing models before deciding on their relative values. Guidelines have been developed to evaluate nursing models and theories by a number of nursing writers (e.g. Meleis 1991, Fawcett 1995). Stevens Barnum (1998) provides comprehensive and easy-to-follow guidelines. However, your feelings about the model are also important and should be part of this evaluation. The guidelines may assist you in choosing a model that fits the needs of your patients/clients or they may guide you in developing your own more appropriate model of nursing. Whether you choose to use guidelines or not, it is worth remembering that we need to appraise all aspects of our practice to ensure that what we are doing is the best and most appropriate for our patients/clients.

2.10 Conclusion

This chapter has briefly explored nursing theory and identified the four main concepts of nursing which are generally accepted as underpinning our values and ideas about care. It has also considered the development of nursing models as a framework for practice. The importance of nurses exploring their own values and beliefs about nursing has been emphasised so that nurses are explicit about their own model of nursing. The use of one model of nursing is considered to be good practice as it is a way of ensuring that nurses work as a team with the same goals. The nursing process was developed as the vehicle for ensuring that nursing theory and the contents of the models are put into practice. Although nursing theory, models and process are widely accepted, the evidence-base for these practices is not always clear as they have not been properly researched. Nonetheless, they are accepted parts of nursing which we need to know about so that we can use them effectively or dismiss them having critically appraised their value to us. The result may be that we create and publish our own theory and model of nursing which is better tailored to the practice setting in which we carry out our caring work.

SELF-EVALUATION

And, finally, your chance to revise what you have learnt from this chapter

1. What are the four main concepts in nursing which underpin nursing theory?
2. Define the term 'nursing model'?
3. What are the five steps of the nursing process?
4. How do nursing theory, nursing models and the nursing process relate?
5. Describe the medical model and how it differs to nursing models?
6. Summarise Roper, Logan and Tierney's activities of living model and identify the 12 activities of daily living.
7. Summarise Roy's adaptation model for nursing.

References

Aggleton, P. and Chambers, H. (2000) *Nursing Models and Nursing Practice* (Second edition). Macmillan, Basingstoke.

Andrews, H. and Roy, C. (1997) *The Roy Adaptation Model.* Appleton and Lange, Norwalk.

Capra, F. (1982) *The Turning Point: Science, Society and the Rising Culture.* Fontana, London.

Chinn, P. and Jacobs, M. (1983) *Theory and Nursing: A Systematic Approach.* Mosby, St Louis.

Christenson, P. and Kenney, J. (1990) *Nursing Process: Application of Conceptual Models.* Mosby, St Louis.

Christenson, P. and Kenney, J. (1995) *Nursing Process: Application of Conceptual Models* (Fourth edition). Mosby, St Louis.

Copernicus, N. (1995) *On the Revolutions of Heavenly Spheres* (Great Minds Series). Prometheus Books, Essex.

Dickoff, J., Weidenbach, E., and James, P. (1968) Theory in a practice discipline. *Nursing Research* 17(5): 415–435.

Downer, P. (2002) Nursing theory and nursing care. In: Kenworthy, N., Snowley, G., and Gilling, C. (eds) *Common Foundation Studies in Nursing.* Churchill Livingstone, London.

Fawcett, J. (1984) The metaparadigm of nursing: Present status and future refinements. *Image* 16(3): 84–89.

Fawcett, J. (1995) *Analysis and Evaluation of Conceptual Models of Nursing.* Davis, Philadelphia.

Fawcett, J. and Downs, F. (1986) *The Relationship of Theory and Research.* Appleton-Century-Crofts, Norwalk.

Fraser, M. (1996) *Conceptual Nursing in Practice: A Research-based Approach* (Second edition). Chapman and Hall, London.

Greenwood, J. (2002) Nursing theory: Its nature and purpose. In: Daly, J., Speedy, S., Jackson, D., and Darbyshire, P. (eds) *Contexts of Nursing: An Introduction*. Blackwell, Oxford.

Helson, H. (1964) *Adaptation Level Theory*. Harper and Row, New York.

Henderson, V. (1966) *The Nature of Nursing: A Definition and its Implications for Practice, Research and Education*. Macmillan, New York.

Jasper, M. (2002) Challenges to professional practice. In: Hogston, R. and Simpson, P. (eds) *Foundations in Nursing Practice: Making a Difference*. Palgrave, Basingstoke.

Johns, C. (1994) *The Burford NDU Model: Caring in Practice*. Blackwell Science, London.

Kershaw, B. and Price, B. (1993) *The Riehl Interaction Model in Action*. Palgrave Macmillan, Basingstoke.

King, I. (1981) *A Theory for Nursing: Systems, Concepts, Process*. Wiley, New York.

Leddy, S. and Pepper, J. (1998) *Conceptual Basis of Professional Nursing* (Fourth edition). Lippincott, Philadelphia.

Maslow, A. (1954) *Motivation and Personality*. Harper and Row, New York.

Meleis, A. (1991) *Theoretical Nursing: Development and Progress*. Lippincott, Philadelphia.

Murphy, M., Cooney, A., Casey, D., Connor, M., O'Connor, J., and Dineen, B. (2000) The Roper, Logan and Tierney (1996) model: Perceptions and operationalization of the model in psychiatric nursing within a health board in Ireland. *Journal of Advanced Nursing* 31(6): 1333–1341.

Neuman, B. (1995) *The Neuman Systems Model* (Third edition). Appleton and Lange, Connecticut.

Neuman, B. and Fawcett, J. (2001) *The Neuman Systems Model*. Prentice Hall, New Jersey.

Orem, D. (1995) *Nursing: Concepts of Practice*. Mosby, St Louis.

Parse, R. (1981) *Man-Living-Health: A Theory of Nursing*. Wiley, New York.

Paul, C. and Reeves, J. (1995) An overview of the nursing process. In: George, J. (ed.) *Nursing Theories: The Base for Professional Nursing Practice* (Fourth edition). Appleton and Lange, Connecticut.

Pearson, A., Vaughan, B., and Fitzgerald, M. (2005) *Nursing Models for Practice* (Third edition). Butterworth Heinemann, Oxford.

Peplau, H. (1952) *Interpersonal Relations in Nursing*. Putnam's Sons, New York.

Rambo, B. (1984) *Adaptation Nursing: Assessment and Intervention*. WB Saunders, Philadelphia.

Riehl, J. and Roy, C. (1980) *Conceptual Models for Nursing Practice* (Second edition). Appleton-Century-Crofts, Norwalk.

Roper, N. (1976) *Clinical Experience in Nurse Education*. Churchill Livingstone, Edinburgh.

Roper, N., Logan, W., and Tierney, A. (1980) *The Elements of Nursing*. Churchill Livingstone, Edinburgh.

Roper, N., Logan, W., Tierney, A., and Holland, K. (2004) *Applying the Roper-Logan-Tierney Model in Practice: Elements of Nursing*. Churchill Livingstone, London.

Rose, P. and Marks-Maran, D. (1997) A new view of nursing: Turning the cube. In Marks-Maran, D. and Rose, P. (eds) *Reconstructing Nursing: Beyond Art and Science. Baillière Tindall, London*.

Roy, C. (1984) *Introduction to Nursing: An Adaptation Model*. Prentice Hall, New Jersey.

Simpson, H. (1991) *Peplau's Model in Action*. Macmillan, Basingstoke.

Stevens Barnum, B. (1998) *Nursing Theory: Analysis, Application, Evaluation* (Fifth edition). Lippincott, Philadelphia.

Thibodeau, J. (1983) *Nursing Models: Analysis and Evaluation*. Wadsworth Health Sciences Division, Monterey.

Visintainer, M. (1986) The nature of knowledge and theory in nursing. *Image* 2: 32–38.

von Bertalanffy, L. (1968) *General Systems Theory*. Brazillier, New York.

Walker, L. and Avant, K. (1996) *Strategies for Theory Construction in Nursing* (Third edition). Appleton and Lang, Norwalk.

Walsh, M. (1989) *Nursing Rituals, Research and Rational Actions*. Heinemann Nursing, Oxford.

Walsh, M. (1998) *Models and Critical Pathways in Clinical Nursing: Conceptual Frameworks for Care Planning*. Baillière Tindall, London.

Yura, H. and Walsh, M. (1967) *The Nursing Process*. Appleton-Century-Crofts, Norwalk.

📖 Suggested reading

Aggleton, P. and Chambers, H. (2000) *Nursing Models and Nursing Practice* (Second edition). Macmillan, Basingstoke.

This book contains an overview of the main models of nursing that are used in practice.

Pearson, A., Vaughan, B., and Fitzgerald, M. (2005) *Nursing Models for Practice* (Third edition). Butterworth Heinemann, Oxford.

This book contains an overview of the main models of nursing that are used in practice. It contains more detail about the origins of nursing models, how to evaluate them and how to choose one. It is also more up to date.

Roper, N., Logan, W., Tierney, A., and Holland, K. (2004) *Applying the Roper-Logan-Tierney Model in Practice: Elements of Nursing.* Churchill Livingstone, London.

This is a useful book to consult to learn about the elements that constitute nursing, to see how a model is constructed and explore how it can be used in practice. It is worthwhile reviewing this book even if you do not think it is a model that you would choose to use as it provides a view about nursing that is practised by many nurses in the United Kingdom.

Learning Through Experience: Reflection and Reflective Practice

3

Chris Bailey

LEARNING OUTCOMES

This chapter should enable you to

- Identify important milestones in the development of our understanding of reflection

- Describe what happens when we reflect

- Identify some important theories or 'models' of reflection

- Discuss how reflection can be used in and contribute to practice

3.1 Introduction

In this chapter, some important milestones in the development of our understanding of reflection are described, and some of the possible applications of reflection to nursing practice are discussed. One particular focus is the contribution of the American philosopher John Dewey, whom many acknowledge as having set out the main principles underlying what we now think of as reflection and reflective practice. Dewey has perhaps contributed more than anyone else to our understanding of the *thought* processes involved in *reflection* (Dewey 1933). Other important contributions to our knowledge of reflection are also discussed, including the work of those with a particular interest in the educational applications of reflection, such as Mezirow (Mezirow and Associates 1990), Kolb and Fry (Cooper 1975, Kolb 1984), Boud *et al.* (1985), Gibbs (1988), Schön (1987), and Johns (2002). Particular attention is drawn to Boud *et al.*'s description of the processes of reflection, including their emphasis on the role of feelings; Chris Johns's work is used to provide an example of how the principles of reflection can be applied in practice as a means of taking action to increase effectiveness. Overall, the purpose of the chapter is to identify important sources of information about reflection, give a summary of some of the theory that underpins it and to suggest some of its applications in nursing practice. The literature on reflection and reflective practice is very extensive indeed, and the hope is that this chapter will provide a useful introduction and stepping-off point for exploring the topic in more detail.

3.2 The nature of reflection

Where does 'reflection' come from?

For many, John Dewey (1859–1952) is one of the most influential figures in the history of what has been written and said about reflection. Dewey, an American philosopher whose work has made an important contribution to educational theory, believed that reflection is about how we *think*, and that *reflective* thinking is a *better* way of thinking (Dewey 1933). Reflective thinking, according to Dewey, means turning a subject over in the mind and giving it serious consideration. Reflective thought is coherent, orderly and logical. It is, says Dewey, thinking something *out*: in other words, there is 'an entanglement to be straightened out, something obscure to be cleared up through the application of thought' (Dewey 1933: 6). So reflection, in Dewey's sense, is neither haphazard nor random. It is thinking with a purpose:

> Active, persistent, and careful consideration of any belief or . . . knowledge in the light of the grounds that support it and the further conclusions towards which it tends constitutes reflective thought.
>
> (Dewey 1933: 9)

By this, Dewey means that reflective thought depends on careful study, reasoning, examination, scrutiny and inquiry; it involves carefully weighing the pros and cons and establishing a firm basis of evidence for what we believe. It is not only a very careful process, it also leads us to think about what the consequences or implications of a particular series of ideas or thoughts might be. So reflection can mean looking forwards, following a chain of thought and thinking ahead.

In *How We Think* (Dewey 1933), Dewey identifies two phases of reflective thinking. First, a state of doubt, hesitation or perplexity (this is where thinking originates); and second, an act of searching, hunting or inquiring in order to resolve doubt or settle uncertainty. To illustrate this, he uses the example of a man who comes to a branching of the road, but does not know which of the two branches he should take, and is therefore hesitant and perplexed. To proceed, the man must find a way of knowing which way is the right way. He must, says Dewey, consider the facts, carefully scrutinise his situation and look for evidence that will tell him which way to go. In a sense, the man is searching for a kind of map to guide him, and reflection is what he uses to discover the facts that will provide him with this. If there is no suggestion of a problem to be solved, says Dewey, our thoughts proceed at random; but if we encounter a question to be answered, or an ambiguity to be resolved, we need to think *reflectively*.

ACTIVITY 3.1

Can you think of an example from practice in which you have had to decide between two alternatives? How could you apply Dewey's idea of reflective thinking to help you resolve your dilemma?

Dewey makes a series of points about reflective thinking that give it a distinctly modern feel, especially in relation to what we now think of, particularly in the health care professions, as *reflective practice*. In *How We Think*, Dewey points out that reflective thinking frees us from impulsive or routine activity, and enables us to know what we are doing while we are doing it. This is an important part of being the kind of practitioner who is critically aware and accountable for his or her actions, and takes us forward to more recent writing that emphasises the value of reflection as a means of overcoming ritual or habitualized practice. Taylor (2000: 43) has described how work can

> become entrenched in routines and habits such as make the beds, do the sponges, showers and baths, check on fluid and food intake.

She explains how

> Daily habits and routines serve their purposes because they get the essential work done, but they can also become a source of practical and emotional numbness, in that the doing of tasks becomes paramount and the people receiving the care become secondary considerations ... Daily habits and routine are a rich area for reflection, because they show you why you are practising in taken-for-granted ways and how you might be able to make some changes ...
>
> (Taylor 2000: 34)

Jack Mezirow, who has written extensively on adult education, believes that critical reflection can free us from our habitual ways of thinking and acting.

According to Mezirow (Mezirow and Associates 1990), reflection helps us to correct 'distortions' in our beliefs and errors in our problem solving: it involves thoroughly testing and 'critiquing' the assumptions on which our beliefs are built in order to move beyond ways of understanding things that have become ingrained or taken-for-granted. What we perceive (and do not perceive), says Mezirow, is greatly influenced by our expectations – by what we are used to. So in order to move on to new perceptions and new understandings, we need to address the possibility that we see, feel or think in a certain way partly because we have stopped questioning our assumptions. Mezirow is clear that acting or doing something in a *reflective* way means acting after critically assessing our own assumptions or examining the justification for our beliefs:

Reflection... involves a pause to reassess by asking: What am I doing wrong? The pause may be only a split second in the decision-making process. Reflection may thus be integral to deciding how best to perform or may involve an ex post facto [i.e. retrospective] reassessment.

(Mezirow and Associates 1990: 6)

Reflection, he suggests, is involved when we look back to reassess the effectiveness of the strategies we have used to solve problems:

We look back to check on whether we have identified all the relevant options for action, correctly assessed the consequences of alternative hunches or hypotheses [and] used the best methods of problem solving and used them correctly and carefully... We may also look to make sure our actions have been consistent with our values [and] to see how well we are doing in relation to our goals...

(Mezirow and Associates 1990: 7)

In nursing, Heath (1998) has suggested that practitioners should be encouraged to reflect on their everyday practice to 'surface' their habitual actions, know their strengths and weaknesses, and maintain a necessary awareness of what they do not know; Paget (2001) notes that reflective practice is seen as a positive force in challenging and identifying ritual practice; and Ipperciel (2003) in effect defines *ritualization* as 'going through the moves' without reflecting. Kim (1999) has described a process of 'critical reflective inquiry', comprising 'descriptive', 'reflective', and 'critical/emancipatory' phases, which, she says, can help practitioners to avoid ritualization and promote learning.

ACTIVITY 3.2

Draw up a shortlist of 'ritual' or 'habitualized' ways of doing things from your own experience of practice. If you find it difficult to think of any, look again at what Taylor (2000) says about daily habits and routines, above. See if you can justify 'daily habits and routines'. Can you think of a better way? On the other hand, can you think of any routines or rituals that make a positive contribution?

According to Dewey, when a difficult or perplexing situation arises, we can either try to avoid it by escaping or retreating from it, or we can face it and try to engage with it. Reflection begins when we commit ourselves to addressing a problematic or perplexing set of circumstances in an engaged way. If we think back to the example of the man who comes to a fork in the road, we can see that for Dewey, reflection is very much about gathering the relevant 'facts' to help us resolve the situation we are faced with. Gathering 'the facts of the case' means *observing* things very carefully to establish the facts, and also using recollection and past experience to help us to identify additional relevant material. Alongside 'gathering the facts', reflection also includes what Dewey calls *suggestions*. *Suggestions* in this sense are possible solutions to the problem we are facing, and reflection involves taking a possible solution and testing it against the facts to see how effective it might actually be. Often, trying out a possible solution in this way will lead to new observations and stimulate further recollections of past experiences, and these can be used in turn to generate more and better solutions until, finally, we have something that addresses the problem in front of us in a satisfactory way. Later writers, particularly those with a background in education, have developed guidelines for reflection that help us to see some of what Dewey had in mind more clearly. Gibbs (1988), for example, developed the simplified idea of a 'reflective cycle' to support learning in practice.

For Dewey, the confused or perplexing situation that is, potentially, the focus of reflection or reflective thought is, more accurately, a *pre*-reflective state of affairs. This *pre-reflective* situation sets us the question that reflection has to answer. There is also, says Dewey, a *post*-reflective situation that occurs when those things that were initially confusing, perplexing or problematic have been resolved through the process of reflection. In between these two states of affairs are five 'phases' of reflective thought (Dewey 1933) (see Box 3.1).

BOX 3.1 Phases of reflective thought

- Suggestions
- Intellectualization
- Hypotheses
- Reasoning
- Testing

Source: Dewey (1933).

In the first of these phases *suggestions* are put forward. This, Dewey argues, is the mind anticipating possible solutions: addressing an uncertain situation reflectively means that instead of acting straightaway, we consider potential ways of responding, or *suggestions*, instead.

In the second phase, says Dewey, we take the difficulty or confusion we are faced with and turn it from a *feeling* that something is not quite right, or that something is out of place, into a definite *problem* to be solved or question to be answered. Dewey calls this phase 'intellectualization'. Reflection is easier if, instead of having to contend with a generally confusing and puzzling set of circumstances, we can pinpoint precisely what the main issue really is. We need to know exactly what the problem or question we are dealing with is before we can start to think about what the solution or answer might be.

The third phase of reflective thought, according to Dewey, involves turning *suggestions*, or more or less spontaneous ideas about what to do, into *hypotheses*. This means taking a suggestion, which is a bit like a guess about how we might resolve a difficult or perplexing set of circumstances, and developing it, through careful observation and consideration of the evidence, into a firmer, clearer idea of what the precise problem is and what the solution might be. We can use hypotheses as preliminary or tentative solutions in situations that raise questions in our minds. Although hypotheses do not finally commit us to a particular course of action or definite conclusion, we can use them as a kind of working model of how to resolve something confusing or perplexing, and as a guide for our investigations, observations and gathering of further 'data' or 'facts'. This in turn will help us to decide whether our *hypothesis* or *working model* is reliable enough to be trusted and followed through.

Dewey's fourth phase of reflection is *reasoning*: reasoning in this sense means exploring the *implications* of what we know about something already, or seeing how one idea leads to another. The fifth and final stage, involves testing proposed solutions, or hypotheses, in practice. This is a means of demonstrating that the ideas we have developed to resolve the difficulties, uncertainties or questions that have challenged us actually work out in reality. Testing our ideas in this way takes us past the tentative 'hypothesis' or 'working model' stage. Naturally, Dewey wasn't specifically thinking of reflective thinking as one of the skills we need as health care professionals, and his examples of 'testing' ideas in practice do not involve *people*. Having reflected on some issue from caring practice and concluded, perhaps, that a certain course of action is warranted, we still need to proceed in a way that takes full account of ethical and professional codes of conduct. Indeed, the importance of skilled *guidance* from an experienced and competent colleague is clearly emphasised in some current models of reflective practice (see, for example, Johns 2002).

Dewey's view of reflection is more systematic and much more impersonal than the one most of us are familiar with today. As he quite clearly states, for him *reflection* is a way of *thinking*, and more precisely, a way of solving problems or resolving uncertainty. His description of reflective thinking emphasizes a rational, objective approach that focuses on the 'facts of the matter' and leaves out much of the *emotional* side of reflection. To health care professionals who have grown up with more recent theories and models of reflection, this might seem like missing the point. A lot of what we learn about reflection today (see, for example, Boud *et al.* 1985, Johns 2002) emphasises the importance in reflection of understanding how a situation makes us *feel*. But Dewey is more concerned with setting out a precise method for thinking that will help us to focus on problems and their solutions. Although this might not seem like 'reflection' to us now, there is, in any process of reflection, a strong component of clear or logical thinking, and this is what Dewey's work helps us to see. In fact, today we might struggle with the idea of reflection precisely because it seems so fluid and intangible. Coming to an understanding that to be able to *reflect* effectively, we usually need to know how to *think* clearly and rationally *first*, tells us a lot about the kind of skills we need to develop in order to become reflective practitioners.

ACTIVITY 3.3

Think about what you already know about 'reflection' and 'reflective practice'. In what way is this different to Dewey's description of 'reflective thinking'? How can Dewey's 'objective' approach to reflection help us to understand what kind of skills are involved in 'reflection' and 'reflective practice'?

3.3 Models of reflection

Learning from experience

Today, reflection is thought of as an essential part of professional practice. A key part of *reflective practice* and being a *reflective practitioner* is knowing how to learn from our experiences. Indeed, experience can be thought of as the starting point for learning (Jasper 2003). Modern writers emphasise the importance of thinking about our experiences, in other words about what happens to us, more explicitly than Dewey does; and the idea that reflection is a way of *learning* from what happens to us has more or less taken over from the idea that reflection is a way of *thinking* about things. But Dewey himself uses examples that show that finding ourselves in perplexing situations can stimulate reflection. For him too, reflection is often rooted in our day-to-day experiences. Dewey is also clear that solving a problem effectively through reflection has implications for the next time we are faced with a problem: in other words, we *learn* things from one episode of reflection that may have a bearing on situations in the future. And today, reflection is still thought of as involving the analytical skills we need to decide what to do in the situations we face in clinical practice (Jasper 2003). The modern view of reflection does not place as much emphasis as Dewey does on its being stimulated by some kind of *problem*. Reflection is often thought of now as something we can apply to almost any experience in order to stimulate learning. As Bulman and Schutz (2004: 4) put it, reflection in nursing is about

> reviewing experience from practice so that it can be described, analysed, evaluated and consequently used to inform and change future practice.

David Kolb and Ronald Fry are well known for their description of a model of learning from experience, or *experiential* learning (see Cooper 1975, Chapter 3), that is often used to guide reflection and reflective practice. A *model* in this sense is a representation of something real; it is a *descriptive picture* of a concept or experience, for example, that is close enough to the real thing to help us understand what is involved in that experience (see Pearson *et al.* 1996).

According to Kolb and Fry, learning, change and personal growth are facilitated by an integrated process:

1. here-and-now experience

followed by:

2. collection of information about the experience

3. analysis of information

4. modification of behaviour

This process can also be shown as a diagram (Figure 3.1):

Learning takes place, say Kolb and Fry, when we apply *cognitive* skills such as questioning or analytical thinking to our immediate, emotional experience in a way that changes our understanding of that experience. New knowledge is achieved through the interaction of the four different aspects of the experiential learning model, so in order to learn effectively, we need to bring together *experience, reflection* and *observation, abstract conceptualization* and *active experimentation.* Learning takes place when we

a) involve ourselves fully, openly and without bias in new experiences

b) reflect on and observe experiences from many perspectives

c) use concepts and ideas to develop potential explanations or theories about experiences

d) use explanations or theories to make decisions and solve problems.

(Cooper 1975: 35–36)

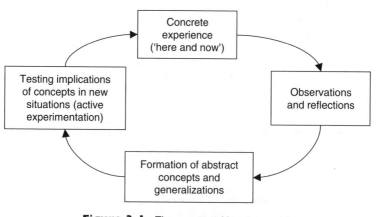

Figure 3.1 The experiential learning model.
Source: Adapted from Cooper (1975).

So, learning is about being *active* (e.g. by testing our theories in practice) as well as being *reflective* (e.g. by interpreting or considering a situation from different perspectives), and about being fully *involved* in an experience as well as being detached and analytical. Kolb and Fry, who are themselves building on theories developed by the psychologist Kurt Lewin (see, for example, Lewin 1951), help us both to pinpoint the role of reflection in the learning process and to identify experience as the starting point for learning.

Graham Gibbs (1988) applies Kolb's experiential learning theory to explain how we might 'learn by doing'. He uses a simplified version of Kolb's experiential learning model to make his point:

In the example he uses to illustrate the process of learning by doing, or experiential learning (Figure 3.2), Gibbs describes how a 'trainee' nurse might begin to (1) learn a clinical skill through supervised practice (e.g. in a clinical skills lab), (2) be encouraged to reflect by being asked how the experience felt, and how things might have been done differently, (3) then explore the evidence base underpinning the skill, and (4) finally begin to put the skill into practice in real situations. Whilst Gibbs' example and the larger work in which it appears throw important light on the principles of experiential learning, the example itself now seems out of date in terms of its description of nursing education and its depiction of approved practices. It refers to 'lifting' a patient, for example, rather than 'moving and handling', and does not refer to the importance of continuing supervision in practice and the formal demonstration of competence by learners. Nevertheless, as Jasper (2003: 78) points out, Gibbs' framework has 'achieved the status of a seminal theory' in reflective practice, and is frequently referred to and drawn upon in textbooks on reflective practice published in recent years.

David Boud, Rosemary Keogh and David Walker have also made an important contribution to our understanding of how reflection plays a key role in turning *experience* into *learning* (see Boud *et al.* 1985). Like Kolb and Fry, they emphasise this connection: reflection is about turning experience into learning, making the most of the situations we find ourselves in and applying our experiences in new contexts. However, they also recognize that Kolb and Fry are not particularly clear about what *reflection* actually is. One of the most helpful things about Boud *et al.*'s (1985) work is that it helps us to focus on what is going on, so to speak, when we reflect on something. When we think of reflection, they say, we usually imagine 'thinking quietly, mulling over events in our mind

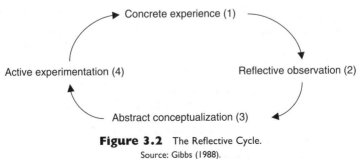

Figure 3.2 The Reflective Cycle.
Source: Gibbs (1988).
Reproduced with permission from Oxford Brookes University.

or making sense of experiences we have had'; perhaps, they say, we could think (metaphorically speaking) of carrying out a 'post-mortem' to help us understand what it means to reflect on a situation we have been in or on something that has happened to us (Boud *et al.* 1985: 8). Experience, particularly in an area that is challenging or unfamiliar (like our clinical practice, for example), can be quite intense and absorbing; it may involve assimilating all sorts of new information, and we may be so immersed in events that we have to draw back from them in order to make sense of them. We may need to keep a record of important events and our thoughts and feelings about them.

According to Boud *et al.* (1985), before we can begin to make sense of our experiences, before we can get a clear picture of what our experiences can teach us, we must first be able to *describe* our experiences and the attitudes and emotions that accompany them. Like Dewey (1933), Boud *et al.* (1985) are clear that reflection is not a kind of day-dreaming: it is something we do with a definite goal or purpose in mind. It is 'goal-directed', focused on learning, understanding or making sense of something better than we did before. What we learn in one situation through reflection we take with us into future experiences as a guide and stimulus to improve performance.

Boud *et al.* (1985) made an important contribution to our thinking about reflection by identifying the importance of *feelings*. *Negative* feelings (particularly about ourselves) are a barrier to learning; *positive* feelings, on the other hand, spur us on and sustain our enthusiasm for learning. Making sense of how an experience or situation makes us feel is a vital part of reflection and is therefore also an essential part of learning from experience. Their model of reflection in learning includes both *experience* (which covers the whole of what we think, feel, and do in response to an event or situation) and reflection *upon* experience. The kind of event or situation they have in mind might be something like a lecture or a workshop, something that happens in practice or just something that happens as part of day-to-day life; it might be an event that takes place in the world around us or it might be something that happens inside us (Boud *et al.* 1985: 18–19).

ACTIVITY 3.4

Think of a situation or event (e.g. something you have heard in a lecture or workshop that has stuck in your mind, or something that has caught your attention or interest in practice). Try to 'mull it over'. Write a detailed description of your experience (you can use notes and jottings), including your thoughts and feelings, what you did, and why. It may be the first time you have thought of the situation in this way. What new light have you been able to throw on it?

Reflection, say Boud *et al.* (1985), is the process involved in *recapturing* our experience, *mulling* it *over* and *evaluating* it; and it is this process that is important in learning. Like Dewey and others (see, for example, Atkins and Murphy 1993), they see reflection as arising out of a sense of discomfort or perplexity; but it can also be the result of more of a positive state of mind – the kind we experience, for example, after successfully accomplishing a difficult task. The experience of successfully accomplishing one thing may, they say, lead us to reflect on and re-evaluate any number of other challenges or issues, and lead to new thoughts and plans for tackling them. So the starting point for reflection, according to Boud *et al.*'s (1985) model, is *experience*, and they are very clear that this means the whole of our response to an event or situation – our thoughts, feelings and actions. We *reflect* by applying certain processes to our experience or experience*s*, and this means focusing on the totality of our response to key events. Like Dewey (1933), Boud *et al.* (1985) regard careful scrutiny of the evidence we can find for interpreting events in a particular way as one of the skills essential to successful reflection; but, unlike Dewey, they emphasise that exploring the feelings aroused in us by events and situations is also a fundamental part of reflection, and just as essential to the process of learning from experience.

Helpfully, Boud, Keogh and Walker set out to take the learner's perspective and provide quite a detailed account of processes for enhancing reflection. They stress the importance of having time after important experiences to 'debrief' and reflect, and suggest that reflection can be facilitated by keeping a diary of our reactions to events. Having a model of reflection helps us to ensure that reflection becomes a planned part of our learning experiences. The model they suggest has three main components: experience, reflective processes and outcomes (Figure 3.3).

Experience (or experiences) forms the first component, and by this Boud *et al.* (1985) mean the totality of our response to a situation or event: our behaviour, ideas and feelings. Experience is the foundation of reflection because it is the raw material, so to speak, that we apply reflective processes to in order to stimulate new understanding, new perspectives or new plans of action. 'Reflective processes' form the second component of the model. The reflective process begins when we 'return' to or recollect our experience (the lecture, the workshop, the key event in our practice or our day-to-day life and so on) with the intention of 'unpacking' it:

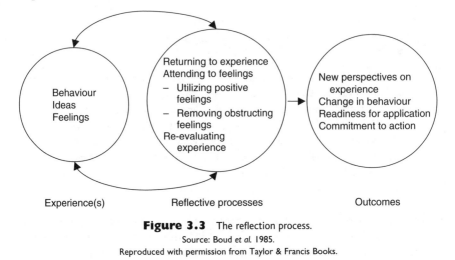

Figure 3.3 The reflection process.
Source: Boud *et al.* 1985.
Reproduced with permission from Taylor & Francis Books.

picking out and putting a name to all the different emotions, ideas, decisions and actions we were part of. We can think of this as 'replaying' the experience, and all our complex reactions to it, in our mind's eye, so that we can reconsider it and re-examine it 'afresh' from a variety of different perspectives (Boud *et al.* 1985: 27–28). Reflection also means 'attending' to our feelings. In particular, we can use positive feelings about our experience as a guide to what *worked* for us, as an indication of those things about our experience that might repay more careful and detailed exploration (not forgetting that we need to explore *critically*, with an awareness of the importance of finding good reasons for concluding that this or that part of a situation went *well*). We also, say Boud *et al.* (1985), need to remove 'obstructing' feelings, by which they mean, for example, that certain aspects of our recollections of experience may be embarrassing or awkward. To understand the experience better, we might need to think about what made things embarrassing for us and overcome that feeling, perhaps by seeing the humorous side or by sharing things with others that we trust and feel comfortable with.

ACTIVITY 3.5

Can you think of a situation in which you felt that things went well for you? What reasons in particular do you have for this positive feeling? Was there anything you felt slight awkward about that you saw in a different light when you had talked it over with friends or colleagues? How did talking things over help?

Finally, reflection is about *re-evaluating* experience. We can gain new insight into our experiences once we have carefully analysed and explored what was positive about them (as well as what was uncomfortable about them). This may involve linking (or *integrating*) new insights we have gained with knowledge we have already accumulated from past experiences, and following through the implications of what we have learned and what has changed in our outlook for our future plans and actions. In a way, say Boud *et al.* (1985), *re-evaluating* experience means *rehearsing* what we might do in future situations in the light of our reflection on current events, with a view to picking out the strengths (and identifying any weaknesses) in our new plans and strategies.

ACTIVITY 3.6

Think of an experience (event or situation) that has helped you to plan for the future (i.e. helped you to change the way you do things). Make a list of the mental 'rehearsals' you went through (the 'what-will-happen-ifs') before you tackled the new situation. What stuck with you most from the initial experience?

Reflection is not an end in itself: it prepares us for future experience (events and situations). In recognition of this, the third component of Boud *et al.*'s (1985) model of reflection highlights the *outcomes* of reflection, which can include new ways of doing things, new ways of seeing issues, new skills and new problem-solving strategies (Boud *et al.* 1985: 34). Familiarity with reflective processes not only helps us to *learn*, it also helps us to *learn how* to learn. Skilful handling of reflective processes is, in effect, the expertise we use to manage the process of learning itself – specifically, learning that not only increases our store of information but also changes, and deepens, our overall view of ourselves, our world (professional and day-to-day) and our ability and commitment to act within that world. Putting new ideas or solutions into practice is not at all a simple matter. It takes, say Boud *et al.* (1985), a positive attitude, and this is one reason why it is important when reflecting on experience to build on positive feelings associated with what we have done well, and to see our way through or 'transform' feelings of awkwardness arising from aspects of situations we have found difficult to handle. For many, this requires sensitive and skilful support, and may mean that reflection is most constructive when it includes an element of guidance or supervision (see Johns 2002).

3.4 Reflective practice

Guided or structured reflection

Although, as Boud *et al.* (1985) point out, individuals can follow many of the processes of reflection through for themselves, there is only so much that we can do alone. Chris Johns has, over many years, developed a framework for *guided reflection* that employs a form of supervision to facilitate the process of learning from experience. Guided reflection, he says, is 'a process of self-inquiry to enable the practitioner to realise desirable and effective practice' (Johns 2002: 3); it is especially useful, he believes, as a way of learning about the 'messy and confusing problems' (see Schön 1987) that often preoccupy us if we are involved in particularly 'human' situations.

ACTIVITY 3.7

You may have experienced something similar to 'guided reflection' yourself, either through your work with your mentor in practice, or through clinical supervision. Think about how your mentor or supervisor has helped you to learn. What has your mentor or supervisor done that has helped you to reflect on practice? What kind of questions have they asked you to help you to look back on your experiences and understand them more fully?

Donald Schön is famous for writing about the idea of 'reflection-in-action'. He believes that some of the questions and problems we encounter in practice cannot be addressed simply by applying standard responses from our existing stock of knowledge:

> Often, a problematic situation presents itself as a unique case ... Because the unique case falls outside the categories of existing theory and technique, the practitioner cannot treat it as an instrumental problem to be solved by applying one of the rules in her store of professional knowledge. The case is not 'in the book.' If she is to deal with it competently, she must do so by a kind of improvisation, inventing and testing in the situation strategies of her own devising.
>
> (Schön 1987: 5)

Sometimes, Schön says, we use 'reflection-*in*-action', which happens almost without our knowing it. We reflect 'in the midst' of an action without interrupting it, and our thinking, he says, actually 'reshapes' what we are doing while we are doing it (Schön 1987: 26). Reflection-in-action is not reflection *on* action because reflection *on* action involves thinking back on something we have done in order to understand how our actions contributed to a particular outcome. Generally speaking, therefore, the ways of thinking about reflection currently popular in nursing are closer to reflection *on* action than they are to reflection-*in*-action; but as Schön suggests, reflection-in-action can still be considered an essential part of skilled performance:

> When good jazz musicians improvise together, they ... display reflection-in-action smoothly integrated into ongoing performance.
>
> (Schön 1987: 30)

The purpose of *reflective practice*, according to Johns, is

> to enable the practitioner to access, understand and learn through, his or her lived experiences and, as a consequence, to take congruent action towards developing increasing effectiveness within the context of what is understood as desirable practice.
>
> (Johns 1995: 226)

Essentially, then, it is about achieving the most effective and desirable form of practice we are capable of. In order to do this, we should reflect on our *current* practice, and the best way to do this, Johns believes, is through a *structured*, or *guided*, approach to reflection. So for Johns, reflection involves a partnership between practitioner and supervisor, and may also take the form of *group* reflection. Learning together, rather than alone, can be more *fun*: guided reflection groups, Johns says, are like 'campfire' gatherings, in which people tell stories, reflect on their own 'wisdom as practitioners' and give voice to 'personal knowing, ideas and opinions' (Johns 2002: 3). Such gatherings are an opportunity to talk and think about what we *already* know, with a view to using dialogue and discussion with others to build on and develop our existing knowledge into more *effective*, more *desirable*, ways of doing things. Johns has identified Barbara Carper's fundamental *Ways of Knowing* in nursing (Carper 1978) as a useful framework for exploring and learning from experience (Johns 1995). 'Knowing' is divided into four dimensions that have their own, distinctive characteristics: empirical, ethical, personal and aesthetic. These different points of view can help us, Johns believes, to make sense of the world of practice, and he uses them to develop a model of structured reflection with 'cue questions' that direct us to the different aspects of our experience represented by the four 'ways of knowing': for example, What was I trying to achieve? What were the consequences for the patient, for others, for myself? What internal factors were influencing me? How did my actions match with my beliefs? What would be the consequences of different actions? (Johns 1995: 227). Essentially, this is a way for us to be more confident that when we reflect on our experiences, we are exploring it in all its diversity and complexity. The *empirical* way of knowing, for example, represents the viewpoint of scientific or theoretical knowledge. The *aesthetic* way of knowing, on the other hand, refers to the way that being in situations often involves *interpreting* information in order to understand the meaning of the situation for those involved, and

> envisioning desired outcomes in order to respond with appropriate and skilled action, and subsequently reflecting on whether the outcomes were effectively achieved.
>
> (Johns 1995: 228)

In order to explore and learn from our experiences, we need to be sensitive to as many of their different aspects and dimensions as possible, and Johns' use of Carper's 'ways of knowing' is one way of helping us to do this. In a later work, Johns uses another framework for reflecting on experience that brings together individual and collective, and subjective and objective points of view as a means of integrating different 'views of knowing' (Johns 2002: 6–8).

Guided or structured reflection is a way of making the contradictions between *desirable* practice and *actual* practice more 'visible' and focusing on actions to *resolve* these contradictions (Johns 1995: 226). The trigger for learning, so to speak, is the contradiction between what we *think*, *feel* and *act* about practice and the values we *aspire* to in practice (Johns 2002: 4). Guided reflection, according to Johns, can involve (and in a sense relies upon) an ongoing, sometimes extended relationship between practitioner and supervisor. His work is full of examples of such relationships. In *Guided Reflection* (Johns 2002), Johns refers to a series of 25 guided reflection sessions with one practitioner over a period of 18 months, and suggests that meetings may take place for one hour every four weeks. In *Caitlin's Story* (Johns 1997) he describes how a guided reflection session with Caitlin, a practitioner, focuses on the decision to withdraw steroids from Ray, who has a meningioma and is dying, and on the consequences of this decision for Lucy, Ray's wife, who is not 'coping' with Ray at home. The withdrawal of medication means that Ray must be admitted to hospital, and the key question for the guided reflection session is whether this is something he would have wanted, and how communication skills might be used more effectively to include Ray more fully in decision-making. This can be seen as an illustration of how in guided reflection, dialogue between the practitioner and the supervisor is used as a means of revealing contradictions in practice, and exploring how we can bring 'actual' and 'desirable' practice closer together. Guided reflection, that is to say, is an important avenue for us to explore in our pursuit of better understanding of clinical experience and the development of professional judgement. On a practical level, however, this can only be achieved through a commitment of time and resources: regular meetings and a willingness to listen and ask focused questions about significant experiences, explore relevant research and theory, apply insights gained from reflective sessions in practice, and reflect, in subsequent sessions, on the impact of these (Johns 2002).

ACTIVITY 3.8

Draw up your own list of evidence about the effectiveness of reflection in learning and in developing understanding and judgement in practice. On the basis of your evidence, do you think it is possible to show that reflection has a positive effect on learning and practice?

3.5 Conclusion

There is an important thread running through ideas about reflection and reflective practice that can be traced back at least as far as Dewey: this is that 'reflective' thinking is a *better* way of thinking, and potentially a way of addressing and resolving the problems that confront us, either in practice or in our everyday lives. Another important thread is that we *learn* from being reflective, and that the lessons of one episode of reflection are not lost, but carried forward with us into the future. Reflection is a way of *learning from experience*, and for some, this means that reflection *changes* us, in the sense that it is a process through which our view of the world is progressively shaped and developed. Research evidence of how we learn through experience has been put forward by educational theorists (see, for example, Cooper 1975, Kolb 1984, Mezirow and Associates 1990), though the point has been made that much of our knowledge about reflection remains theoretical (Duke and Appleton 2000). Some writers remain sceptical about the claims made for the various forms of reflection (see, for example, Greenwood 1993, Clinton 1998, Gilbert 2001); others, like Johns, believe that insisting that reflective practice is tested experimentally to demonstrate its effectiveness is missing the point, and that 'narrative' (i.e., people's own *accounts* of reflective practice) adequately demonstrate its efficacy (Johns 2002). This is not a bad debate to have, because in the end, we should always make careful judgements before making the kind of claims that are made about reflection and reflective practice. The only way to decide, though, is to carefully review the evidence for ourselves!

━━━━━━━ **SELF-EVALUATION** ━━━━━━━

?

And, finally, your chance to revise what you have learnt from this chapter

- Describe reflective thinking according to Dewey (1933) and consider how you may apply this to practice.

- Write down the five phases of reflective thought described by Dewey (1933) and explain each of them.

- Draw Kolb and Fry's experiential learning cycle. Think of an example from practice and use this cycle to aid your learning.

- Use Gibbs' (1988) reflective cycle to assist you in reflecting on an incident from practice.

- Describe reflection according to Boud *et al.* (1985) and consider how you might apply this to practice.

- What does Schön (1987) mean by reflection-in-action?

References

Atkins, S. and Murphy, K. (1993) Reflection: A review of the literature. *Journal of Advanced Nursing* 8: 1188–1192.

Boud, D., Keogh, R., and Walker, D. (1985) *Reflection: Turning Experience into Learning.* Routledge Falmer, London.

Bulman, C. and Schutz, S. (2004) *Reflective Practice in Nursing.* Blackwell Publishing, Oxford.

Carper, B. (1978) Fundamental ways of knowing in nursing. *Advances in Nursing Science* 1(1): 13–23.

Clinton, M. (1998) On reflection in action: Unaddressed issues in refocusing the debate on reflective practice. *International Journal of Nursing Practice* 4: 197–202.

Cooper, C.L. (1975) *Theories of Group Processes.* John Wiley and Sons, London.

Dewey, J. (1933) *How We Think: A Restatement of the Relation of Reflective Thinking to the Educative Process.* DC Heath and Company, Lexington, Massachusetts.

Duke, S. and Appleton, J. (2000) The use of reflection in a palliative care programme: A quantitative study of the development of reflective skills over an academic year. *Journal of Advanced Nursing* 32(6): 1557–1568.

Gibbs, G. (1988) *Learning by Doing: A Guide to Teaching and Learning Methods.* Further Education Unit. Oxford Polytechnic (now Oxford Brookes University), Oxford.

Gilbert, T. (2001) Reflective practice and clinical supervision: Meticulous rituals of the confessional. *Journal of Advanced Nursing* 36(2): 199–205.

Greenwood, I. (1993) Reflective practice: A critique of the work of Argyris and Schön. *Journal of Advanced Nursing* 18: 1183–1187.

Heath, H. (1998) Paradigm, dialogues and dogma: Finding a place for research, nursing models and reflective practice. *Journal of Advanced Nursing* 28(2): 288–294.

Ipperciel, D. (2003) Dialogue and decision in a moral context. *Nursing Philosophy* 4: 211–221.

Jasper, M. (2003) *Beginning Reflective Practice.* Nelson Thornes, Cheltenham.

Johns, C. (1995) Framing learning through reflection within Carper's fundamental ways of knowing in nursing. *Journal of Advanced Nursing* 22: 226–234.

Johns, C. (1997) Catlin's story – realizing caring within everyday practice through guided reflections. *International Journal for Human Caring* 1(2): 33–39.

Johns, C. (2002) *Guided Reflection: Advancing Practice*. Blackwell Science, Oxford.

Kim, H.S. (1999) Critical reflective inquiry for knowledge development in nursing practice. *Journal of Advanced Nursing* 29(5): 1205–1212.

Kolb, D.A. (1984) *Experiential Learning: Experience as the Source of Learning and Development*. Prentice Hall Inc., Englewood Cliffs, New Jersey.

Lewin, K. (1951) *Field Theory in Social Science*. Harper and Row, New York.

Mezirow, J. and Associates (1990) *Fostering Critical Reflection in Adulthood*. Jossey-Bass Publishers, San Francisco.

Paget, T. (2001) Reflective practice and clinical outcomes: Practitioners' views on how reflective practice has influenced their clinical practice. *Journal of Clinical Nursing* 10: 204–214.

Pearson, A., Vaughan, B., and Fitzgerald, M. (1996) *Nursing Models for Practice*. Butterworth Heinemann, Oxford.

Schön, D.A. (1987) *Educating the Reflective Practitioner*. Jossey-Bass Publishers, San Francisco.

Taylor, B.J. (2000) *Reflective Practice: A Guide for Nurses and Midwives*. Open University Press, Buckingham.

@ Useful websites

http://www.siu.edu/~deweyctr/   The Center for Dewey Studies, Southern Illinois University

http://www.infed.org/   independent website on informal education

📖 Suggested reading

Johns, C. (2000) *Becoming a Reflective Practitioner*. Blackwell Science, London.
This book offers a reflective and holistic approach to clinical nursing, practice development and clinical supervision.

Bulman, C. and Schutz, S. (2004) *Reflective Practice in Nursing*. Blackwell Publishers, London.
This book assumes no prior knowledge of reflection and draws from practice, experience allowing the realities and practicalities of using reflection to be illustrated.

Humanities in Nursing: Exploring Meanings of Illness to Enhance Patient-Centred Care

Janice Brown

CONTENTS

- Distinction between art and science in nursing

- Introduction to the humanities in nursing

- Range of resources for engaging with nursing humanities

- Evidence base for using the nursing humanities to enhance patient-centred care

LEARNING OUTCOMES

This chapter should enable you to

- Appreciate a distinction between the art and science of nursing

- Understand the potential of the 'nursing humanities' for enhancing patient-centred care

- Appreciate the impact of engaging with materials from the nursing humanities

- Identify and discuss the evidence related to engaging with nursing humanities

4.1 Introduction

This chapter explores the potential impact upon caring practices through engaging with narratives from people who have experienced illness and suffering.

These 'narratives' might be presented as novels, poetry or even art, music and film but they all share a common intention: that of expressing the insider perspective of people who have lived and died from illness. Suggesting that we spend time reading poetry and literature might appear an indulgent activity in a health care world of limited resources, objective targets and with the need to be responsive to a plethora of policies. However, growing evidence suggests that engaging with patients' experiences through their stories and other materials can enhance creative thinking and fine-tune our attentiveness to people (Carson 1994), improve our communication skills (Throw and Murray 1991) and develop our understanding of key concepts such as attributes of patient-centred care (Jackson and Sullivan 1999). You may have experienced for yourself how when comparing a novel or a film with a friend, that the two of you may have understood the story in different ways. McAdams (1993) suggests this is the value of stories as they encourage us to think, present us with differing ideas and opinions, allow us to see and possibly to understand better what we might not have seen before.

Theoretical contributions in the field of chronic illness have drawn on patients' perspectives to develop conceptual interpretations. Bury (1982) identifies how chronic illness can be a 'biographical disruption' whereby an illness such as rheumatoid arthritis in the young can undermine their taken-for-granted sense of self and their anticipated future. Charmaz (1983) develops the concept of *loss of self* to describe how illness can change a person. Think of a person with a chronic illness who becomes housebound, socially isolated, physical restricted and a burden to others. If this was a new description of you, do you think you would change how you currently view yourself? These important theoretical concerns, secured through focusing on people's subjective experiences, can offer us an understanding of lay experiences of illness which is in contrast to the normally medically dominant perspective of illness. Modern medicine often objectifies patients (Parsons 1951, Illich 1976), reducing people to body parts with implicit responsibilities to accept medical wisdom rather than as holistic beings with minds, meanings and values of their own to participate in their care.

The practice of nursing takes place within the context of narrative as people relate their stories of illness and suffering. These experiences may be told through tones of sadness, suffering, courage and humour. As people share their stories, rich streams of meanings flow with evidence of endurance, hope, fear and expectation. These unique insights into patients' worlds offer nurses the opportunity to understand more about being human and the importance of care and human interaction through illness. However, learning from these stories requires an open heart and mind, attentive listening and an ability to reflect. If these opportunities are embraced, patients' stories can be a deep seam of knowing to develop our personal knowledge of being human in situations of distress. Integration of this learning into our practice presents possibilities to guide our professional judgement to enhance patient-centred care.

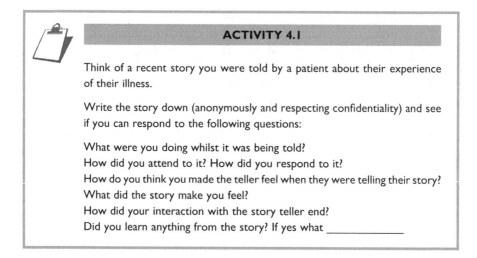

ACTIVITY 4.1

Think of a recent story you were told by a patient about their experience of their illness.

Write the story down (anonymously and respecting confidentiality) and see if you can respond to the following questions:

What were you doing whilst it was being told?
How did you attend to it? How did you respond to it?
How do you think you made the teller feel when they were telling their story?
What did the story make you feel?
How did your interaction with the story teller end?
Did you learn anything from the story? If yes what _____

It can be argued that developing skills to listen and learn from stories is a neglected part of formal nurse education. Learning about reflection is a supportive activity (see Chapter 3) but learning from patients' stories traditionally takes place in the practice setting although this process can be fraught with difficulties. Literature and poetry, however, offer us relatively safe materials to study and learn from human experiences. These materials can 'encourage reflection, promote self-awareness and stimulate debate on difficult issues, for example, death and dying, power and institutionalisation (of patients and staff) and pain' (Robb and Murray 1999: 1182). Literary criticism skills are not essential here but drawing on your skills of reflection is important (Atkins and Murphy 1993) to be able to analyse and synthesize a variety of meanings and to apply this learning into practice. Moyle *et al.* (1995: 961) support the use of literature because 'if nurses are to develop their role of nurturing and caring for sick and healthy people, then they must engage in educational experience and learning which helps to develop insight and understanding further'. This means focusing not only on physical aspects but also on the more personal patient-centred aspects of what it means to be ill.

4.2 Art and science in nursing

There is agreement that the practice, discipline and knowledge base of nursing encompass both artistic and scientific elements (Kitson 1993). A considerable strand of literature exists which exhorts this debate. Science is considered objective, detached, full of doubt, requiring evidence and sceptical. Art is considered a skill, creative, intuitive, subjective, tacit and 'seen' in action rather than documented. Parker (1997: 3) suggests the status of science is still in the ascendancy, 'to the possible detriment of patient-centred humanistic nursing practice'.

If you examine your nurse education programme, you are probably experiencing a predominantly formal delivery through an academic health sciences context with the content mainly based on knowledge emanating from the sciences. The teaching of life sciences is imperative for understanding human physiology and pathology, and that of the social sciences for appreciating how 'individuals interact with each other in society' (Robinson 1992: 60) together with the 'systematic study of people and their behaviour' (Clark 1992: 90). Whilst the importance of scientific and objective knowledge is acknowledged, it can be argued that a dearth of interpretive and subjective forms of knowledge presents dangers for preparing nurses for the reality of practice.

Schön (1987) regards practice as the 'swampy lowlands' of uncertainty because it often confounds factual knowledge and requires interpretation and 'know-how'. Engaging in this uncertain, subjective world requires not only self-awareness and personal knowledge but the willingness and flexibility to understand other people who exist in their own worlds of multiple meanings. As health care professionals, we need to understand and learn about this world as much as the logical, objective world of science.

ACTIVITY 4.2

Think about how your professional education programme is organised.
List out the modules (also called units of learning) you study and find out what is written about the aims of each module.

Which modules would you identify as based on the sciences?
Which modules would you identify as based on a more human focused or interpretive model?

How do you learn to understand what it means to be ill?
How do you learn to be sensitive, connect with a patient, relate to their situation and empathise?

Science and technology have undoubtedly improved the human condition through extending and improving the quality of our lives. The emphasis on securing objective knowledge, the cause and effect of disease and related interventions revolves around patho-physiological aspects of the body and is practiced through the medical disease model. However, privileging the scientific worldview only serves to diminish the subjective side of being human, the world of practice and meanings, of illness and suffering. As Kleinman (1988: xiv) states, the 'One unintended outcome of the modern transformation of the medical care system is that it does just about everything to drive the practitioner's attention away from the experience of illness'.

People who develop illness rely on nurses to harness the benefits of science but they also expect 'human recognition of their suffering' (Charon *et al.* 1995: 599). Fears of losing the balance between science and care have been signposted for some time. Isabel Stewart (1929: 1) stated nursing encompasses and 'mandates a balance of the head, the heart, and the hands or the science, the skill, and the spirit. We have forged ahead in the area of science and technology, but there is fear among us that the spirit becomes dimmer and dimmer with the passage of time'. Privileging one aspect of being human over another or leaving one to chance could have serious implications for recipients and deliverers of health care. Nearly 60 years on, Moyle *et al.* (1995: 961) suggest that in our 'quest for demanding every facet of practice to be scrutinised for conscious explanation to achieve maximum return of efficiency and effectiveness, we are trying to reduce everything to clear reasoned concepts that can be quantifiable and replicated. This results in the human being taking second place to these demands leading to humans being treated as objects rather than subjects'. If the subjective side of illness is not equally promoted then as Moyle *et al.* (1995) state, the art of caring and compassionate awareness of humanity may become neglected.

ACTIVITY 4.3

Consider and write down what you think are the main aspiring attributes of being a nurse. To help in this process, Simone Roach (1992) suggested there are five attributes which she calls the 5C's. They are listed below. You can look up in the literature to see how she described them but see if you can write out your own thoughts first.

Compassion is _____
Competence is _____
Commitment is _____
Communication is _____
Conscience is _____
Can you think of any more _____

We have already seen in Chapter 2 how nursing theories and models (Aggleton and Chalmers 2000) were written to clarify the discipline and practice of nursing. Within these models we can find influences of both science and art. Traditional science disciples, politics, philosophy and economics (Mason and Whitehead 2003) are strong sources of knowledge and there are nursing models which predominantly draw on the sciences (Roy 1976, Orem 1980). Equally there are protagonists who predominantly draw on humanistic and caring knowledge (Paterson and Zderad 1976, Watson 1988, Bishop and Scudder 1991, Parse 1998, Boykin and Schoenhofer 2001) where the emphasis focuses on holism, spirituality, life experiences, personhood, subjectivity, caring, helping and patient-centred practice. We must be cognisant that patients' concerns normally span physical imperatives of relief of pain or treatment of symptoms as well as the need for understanding and effective nurse–patient relationships. However, as nursing claims that its specific domain 'is people's responses to and experience of health, illness, frailty, and disability, in whatever environment or circumstances they find themselves' (Royal College of Nursing 2002: 2), the case is strong for nurses to understand these concepts and appreciate the patient's and family carers' experiences.

ACTIVITY 4.4

It is useful to revise Chapter 2 on nursing models.

Can you remember the four concepts that are part of a nursing model (Fawcett 1984) where each author should state their values and beliefs? What are your underlying values and beliefs of these four concepts?

Try to describe the underlying beliefs of a model related to your field of practice (it might be useful to revisit the book by Aggleton and Chalmers [2000] for this). Does your chosen model reflect the science and art of nursing?

4.3 Humanities in nursing

To rise to the challenge of finding ways to understand patient experiences, an obvious source is to investigate the research literature. There is evidence about the experience of illness, dying trajectories and living with chronic illness (Glaser and Strauss 1968, Fitzpatrick *et al.* 1984, Morse and Johnson 1991, Madjar and Walton 1999, Small and Rhodes 2000). These qualitative studies offer us a glimpse of patients' worlds and how they may differ from the professional world. A study examining quality of life (QOL) in the context of a life-limiting neuro-disability (motor neurone disease) concluded that 'individual QOL appears to be largely independent from physical function in severely ill patients' (Neudert *et al.* 2004: 551) but most dependent on family, friends and their social life. Whilst most health care practitioners operate in the disease or medical model, Neudert's research indicates that patients' illness experiences may actually present a different set of priorities and needs than the disease model advocates. This challenges us to rethink our traditions and demands that we become more in tune with patients' perspectives to support them in meeting their needs.

ACTIVITY 4.5

Think of a patient that you have cared for. Can you imagine their illness journey? What were its key features?

Morse and Johnson (1991: 2) suggest that a comprehensive illness model could provide insights for health care professionals, as well as offering a basis for the planning and implementation of care. But in its absence, we should consider the challenge and impact of seeking insights through studying literature, biographies, film and poetry produced by people who have experienced illness and suffering. William Styron's (1991) offers his first-hand account of depression in *Darkness Visible*; Dave Peltzer's recounts in three books his experiences of being an abused child, *A Child Called It* (1995), *The Lost Boy* (1997) and *A Man Called Dave* (2000) (all in Peltzer 2002). Other sources may be more classical works which have something significant to offer in this field, including John Clare's poetry (much on the experience of depression), C.S. Lewis on bereavement in *A Grief Observed* (Lewis 1961), Mahler's musical 9th symphony on the death of his child and Edvard Munch's series of paintings about death and 'The Sick Child'. Although these are all interpretations about experiences and as we engage with them we add to the interpretive layer, it is what we can learn from them that is important.

The study of these works serves to re-focus the social or *medical* condition in context with the *person* and offers insight into differences in interpretations, values and individual perceptions. This practice has been pursued in medical education in the United States since the 1970s (Charon *et al.* 1995) and more recently in the United Kingdom (Kirklin 2001). The motivation for the rise of the *medical humanities* is parallel to that in nursing. Gogel (1987 cited in Darbyshire 1995: 211) states the importance of medical humanities is to 'celebrate the contextual nature of a text and its possibilities for multiple interpretations and argue that patients coming to health care professionals and care settings need to be approached and similarly understood'. Acknowledgment of the individuality of people is central to Kirklin's (2001: 25) suggestions that two objectives of engaging with the humanities are, first, to encourage the process of reflection (see Chapter 3) so practitioners can engage with their feelings, inclinations, practice and experiences. The second is to allow practitioners to appreciate the experience of illness by patients and their carers.

The term 'nursing humanities' was developed in the mid-1990s (Darbyshire 1995: 211, Moyle *et al.* 1995) to describe the formal use of literature through programmes of learning by nurse educationalists. These courses offered to expose a way of knowing that goes beyond ordinary experience, to foster analytical and creative thinking (Hargrave 1985) and to promote a student's capacity to be a caring practitioner (Darbyshire 1994, Hodges *et al.* 2001). The approach taken in these courses is to question materials, seek puzzles and live with unresolved issues rather then secure final answers. The outcome can be personalised learning (Darbyshire 1995: 215) and contribute to the development of aesthetic and personal knowledge (Carper 1978, see Chapters 1 and 3). This serves to prepare us as practitioners for future situations and increase our capacity for making patient-centred professional judgements.

Let us engage now with some poetry to make our own decisions about the impact of such materials. It is reputedly written by an anonymous woman in an elderly care ward. Read it carefully and make a note of your reaction and any learning points.

Extract from Crabbit Old Woman (anonymous)
(*Found in an elderly woman's locker after she died in hospital*)

> What do you see nurses, what do you see?
> What are you thinking when you are looking at me-
> A crabbit old woman, not very wise.
> Uncertain of habit with far-away eyes.
> Who dribbles her food and makes no reply,
> When you say in a loud voice 'I do wish you'd try'.

Who seems not to notice the things that you do
And is always losing a stocking, a shoe
Who unresisting or not lets you do as you will
With bathing and feeding, the long day to fill.
Is that what you're thinking? Is that what you see?
Then open your eyes nurse, you are not looking at me.
I'll tell you who I am as I sit here so still
As I rise at your bidding and eat at your will.
I'm a small child of ten with a father and mother:
Brothers and sisters who love one another:
A young girl of sixteen with wings on her feet
Dreaming that soon now a lover she'll meet:
A bride soon at twenty my heart gives a leap
Remembering the vows that I promised to keep:
At twenty-five now I have young of my own
Who need me to build a secure happy home
A woman of thirty, my young now grow fast,
Bound to each other with ties that should last.
At forty my young sons now grown, will be gone:
But my man stays beside me to see I don't mourn;
At fifty once more babies play around my knee;
Again we know children, my loved one and me
Dark days are upon me, my husband is dead
I look to the future and shudder with dread.
My young are all busy rearing young of their own.
And I think of the years and the love that I've known.
I'm an old woman now and nature is cruel.
'Tis jest to make old age look like a fool.
The body crumbles, grace and vigour depart.
There is now a stone where I once had a heart.
But inside this old carcass a young girl still dwells
And now and again my battered heart swells.
I remember the joys, I remember the pain,
And I'm loving and living all over again.
And I think of the years all too few – gone too fast
And accept the stark fact that nothing will last.
So open your eyes, nurse, open and see,
Not a crabbit old woman, look closer – see me!

ACTIVITY 4.6

There is a written response by a nurse to this poem. See if you can write your own response to the 'Crabbit Old Woman'.

ACTIVITY 4.7

Having read the poem, describe on paper your feelings and reaction to it. What questions does this poem raise for you? What issues still puzzle you? Can you isolate any new perspectives you may have gained about being elderly or had reinforced that could influence your practice?

To assist in your reflections, Box 4.1 offers an adaptation of Driscoll's (1994) reflective structure as a useful starting guide to explore the nursing humanities. You might like to use this tool to deepen your analysis and synthesis of interpretation.

BOX 4.1 The humanities reflective cycle

What?
What type of story is being expressed? Sad, happy, hopeful, vulnerable . . . ?
What do I feel from this experience?
What message(s) do I understand?
How can I describe the experience that is being expressed to others?

So what?
What do I understand by this experience in relation to me?
What meanings do I interpret in relation to the illness experience?
What meanings do I interpret in relation to the practice of nursing?

Now what?
What have I learnt from this experience?
How (if at all) has the experience changed my thinking?
How (if at all) has the experience changed my personal knowledge?
How might I change/modify my practice as a result of this experience?
What other issues about nursing practice has this reflective exercise raised for me that I would like to further examine through using this approach?

Source: Adapted from Driscoll (1994).

Let us now consider literature. In this section I will offer extracts from five autobiographical novels to explore meanings of illness.

ACTIVITY 4.8

Get a pen and some paper. As you read this next section make notes of your reactions to the quotes but also to the interpretations. Make a particular note of any differences in meaning you make from the extracts.

Ruth Picardie, a young journalist, wrote extensive e-mail messages to friends and articles in the *Observer* newspaper about her experiences of living with breast cancer. They were posthumously published as 'Before I Say Goodbye' (Picardie 1998). Ruth's journalistic flair and humorous writing holds the reader in tears between laughter and sadness simultaneously. Her experiences are far ranging and teach us about the power of the medical profession, taking control through developing her own 'therapies', the denial of death supported through language and the emotional pain of dying.

In one section Ruth reports how she knew her cancer had spread to the brain. When she asks the doctors to scan her head, they delay with awful consequences. She writes, 'if they'd taken me seriously when I first reported the pain in my head, I could have had it all blitzed in one go...it just took me weeks to convince them I needed a CT scan...I think from now on they won't fob me off' (Picardie 1998: 30–31). The doctors' lack of belief in her self-knowledge frustrated and annoyed her but can teach us the significance of professional arrogance and the importance of respecting people's knowledge of themselves.

As medical treatments and therapies became less effective for Ruth she found her own in retail therapy; buying expensive make-up, watching Channel 4's *ER* and *Friends* and eating lots of chocolate. We can learn how she is trying to take control of her life again, to normalize things through 'personal indulgence and escapism' (Picardie 1998: 78). These actions contribute a small sense of victory to her but emphasize how illness provokes people to deal with a range of distresses and 'the practical problems of daily living' (Kleinman 1988: 4).

Ruth initially denied her impending death as 'One way of coping is denial i.e. certainty that you are going to be one of the few that make it' (Picardie 1998: 16–17), although her known odds were 18 per cent for a five-year survival. She observes how health professional language is also in denial writing, 'Cancer is all about fear, secrecy and euphemism – palliative care, advanced disease – all are euphemisms for dying. Oncology is the biggest euphemism in the world' (Picardie 1998: 13). However, death to her meant 'losing the future. I won't be there to clap when my beloved babies learn to write their names; I won't be there to see them learn to swim, or go to school, or play the piano...' (Picardie 1998: 58). Her greatest fear was of loss as after only 33 years of life that 'It's just that I'll miss it so' (Picardie 1998: 59).

As I read Ruth's account, I learnt and questioned more about the place of denial, normality in abnormal conditions, beliefs and practices around dying and the importance of acknowledgment of lives in death. I was concerned about the power of professionals, the dismissal of patients' self-knowledge and the importance of control through 'alternative' therapies. Although Ruth's experiences are personal, her writings offer new ways of thinking about the experience of illness to enhance us to be more in a state of readiness to others.

Four other novels will be touched on with brevity to tease out an insight from each. John Diamond, a *Sunday Times* journalist, had tongue cancer. He explored 'what was it like to be a person with cancer, to deal with the pain and the fear and the anger?' (Diamond 1998: 1). He found cancer medical texts but little about the experience of being a person with cancer, hence his book 'Because cowards get cancer too' (Diamond 1998). Diamond offers particular insight into frustrations of living without speech after a tracheostomy. He writes of his perceived link between communication ability and mental health, 'It was bad enough having a wonky voice but having a wonky voice and sounding like a stupid person was intolerable' (1998: 211).

Dennis Potter offers a positive feature in facing his mortality as he shines with his description of learning the meaning of the 'nowness' of life. He writes that 'the blossom is out in full now . . . and looking at it through the window when I'm writing, I see it is the whitest, frothiest, blossomist blossom that there ever could be, . . . The nowness of everything is absolutely wondrous, and if people could see that' (Potter 1994: 5). This 'nowness' invokes a temporal realization and a fresh perspective on life, a gain when facing one's death but also illustrative of the depth of emotions experienced under duress (see Chapter 6).

Robert McCrum (1998) and Jean-Dominique Bauby (1997) both wrote of their cerebrovascular accidents. Robert was paralysed down one side and temporarily unable to speak but survived. Jean was immobilized and lost all speech but wrote his book through dictating with his eye lashes, only to die just after his book was published.

McCrum writes of the vulnerability of our bodies as, 'The unexpected failure of the body is a shocking catastrophe that threatens the flimsy edifice that we call the "self"' (McCrum 1998: 50). The effects of his disabilities made him realize his change of self as he, 'was no longer the person I'd been twenty-four hours ago' (McCrum 1998: 13). In this condition of vulnerability he describes one nurse as his guardian angel, who 'had a lovely smile and the most gentle manner' (McCrum 1998: 20). However, he also explains how as a passive recipient of care he must 'submit to the experiences' (McCrum 1998: 108), which highlights the theme of power and illustrates the vulnerability of being cared for. Bauby (1997) offers an incident which illustrates differences in perceptions between care professionals and patients. His immobility meant he was introduced to a wheelchair. To the therapist this was a functional achievement, to him it was a disaster, ' "You can handle the wheelchair," said the occupational therapist with a smile intended to make the remark sound like good news, whereas to my ears it had the ring of a life-sentence' (Bauby 1997: 17).

ACTIVITY 4.9

What questions did the extracts raise for you? Did you agree with the interpretations? What puzzling issues did you identify? Did you identify any new perspectives about living with cancer or disability, or meanings of illness? Do you feel motivated to read these texts for yourself in their entirety?

4.4 Resources for studying humanities in nursing

In your own searches for humanities materials you will find a range of literature, poetry and indeed music, art and photography which people have used to express their experiences. One medium may be more preferable to you than another. As Polson and Farmer (2002) highlight the difficulties involved in financing studying humanities in nursing, particularly due to copyright costs, it is prohibitive in this text to add photographs, works of art, and a much wider range of literature and poetry in this chapter. However, Box 4.2 offers a start to your own searching. Web-based resources can be unstable, so use these as only part of your exploration. I hope you find many more.

BOX 4.2 Useful resources to explore the humanities in different modes

Books

De Hennezel, M. (1997) *Intimate Death. How the dying teach us to live* (Trans. Carol Janeway) Little Brown and Company, London.
> This book is written from the perspective of a health professional working in a hospice in France and her encounters with people in their journey towards death.

Lewis, C.S. (1961) *A Grief Observed*. Faber and Faber, London.
> A classic written by C.S. Lewis following the death of his wife.

Reeve, C. (1998) *Still Me*. Arrow Books. London.
> Christopher Reeve's account of living with a broken neck after a horse-riding accident rendered him paraplegic.

Smith, R. (2004) *Amazing Grace: Enjoying Alzheimer's*. Metro Publishing, London.
> A husband's account of looking after his wife with Alzheimer's disease.

Cole, J. (2004) *Still Loves Narrative of Spinal Cord Injury. A Bradford Book.* The MIT Press, London.
> A book reflecting the narratives of 12 people living in a wheelchair following a spinal cord injury 'to listen to their loves as they express them'.

Ulla-Carin Lindquist (2005) *Rowing Without Oars*. John Murray, London.
> This is a personal account of living and dying with motor neurone disease.

Kaysen, S. (1993) *Girl, Interrupted*. Virago Press, London.
> This is an autobiography of a young girl who was committed to a mental institution.

Websites on people's stories of their experiences of illness

http://www.lifechallenges.org
http://www.dipex.org
This is hosted by a charity that funds research to carry out in-depth interviews into patients' experience of health and illness. The aim is to identify the things that matter to people when they have a health problem (e.g. accounts of parents of children with congenital heart disease, epilepsy, hypertension, cancers, etc.).

Films/Videos

Born on the Fourth of July, starring Tom Cruise – the journey of a soldier after serving in Vietnam, adjusting to life in a wheelchair.

A Beautiful Mind, starring Russell Crowe – insight into living with schizophrenia.

Iris, starring Judi Dench – portraying the life of Iris Murdoch and her deterioration through Alzheimer's disease.

BOX 4.2 continued

Art

The following resources take you to websites where you can view specific works of art.

Edward Munch Gallery. Munch has a particular interest in death, with a series of superb paintings and also a famous painting of 'The Sick Child' (1970). http://www.edvard-munch.com/gallery/death/sickChild2.htm

Tate Gallery. This is the email connection to the Tate Gallery, London. I would suggest you specifically view Kossoff's work which offers a vivid sense of human suffering and illustrates his views of the tragic nature of human Existence. http://www.tate.org.uk

Frida Kahlo. Frida's work is particularly interesting in terms of her views on not being able to have children. She was involved in a terrible tram accident in her early twenties when a metal rod pierced her womb. Her expressive portrayal of her own body and its imagery of babies are very powerful. http://members.aol.com/fridanet/kahlo.htm

Damien Hurst and Pharmacy. Highlights perceptions of drugs and pharmacies. http://www.tate.org.uk/pharmacy/

The National Gallery is full of art that has relation to illness – have a browse for yourself but the following sites offer art in this context. Full notes are offered by the gallery for you to appreciate their interpretations. http://www.nationalgallery.org.uk

Photography

A useful text which examines death and offers powerful photographs for our consideration: Bertman, S.L. (1991) *Facing Death: Images, Insights and Interventions*. Taylor and Francis, London.

Music

Much music has been written with a real sense of meaning and experience behind it. You will have your favourites but have you listened to either Mahler's 9th symphony inspired by the last breath of love (his daughters and his impending death) or Sting's – 'Fragile': About the fragility of being human?

4.5 Do the humanities promote person-centred practices?

You should have started to form a view about learning from the nursing humanities and its potential influence on your personal knowledge development and future practice. However, Darbyshire (1995) suggests that it is too simplistic to assume a causal relationship between studying literature and making us more humane practitioners. Merely reading literature does not make us into more compassionate persons. Without a desire, an openness and willingness to learn there may be no effect at all. Indeed Woodcock (1990: 44 cited in Darbyshire 1995: 212) reminds us to remember how '... the Nazi's love of Beethoven taught us that a mere appreciation of art cannot be relied upon to humanise'. We must be mindful of our inherent caring motivations and how the nursing humanities can enhance our understanding and breadth of meanings of illness and keep alive our passion for patient-centred care.

A criticism of the use of the nursing humanities is also its strength. The potential for multiple meanings from stories offers an arbitrary and unscientific approach in that there can be no objective truth. However, the tradition of interpretation (hermeneutics) argues that we are formulating our understanding and meanings all the time as this is how we make sense of our world. Interpretations are based on our previous experiences and interpretations, as this is all we have. In this tradition, the imperative is to keep questioning and exploring. Language dominates our exploration; even though we can experience and understand messages through a wider range of materials beyond words. Posing questions to embrace multiple meanings opens us to possibilities, safeguards us from becoming narrow and blinkered to possibilities. Gadamer (cited in Bleicher 1980: 113) suggests new experiences can be gained through such questioning which leads us to 'now not only know more but to know better'. It is this quest which lies at the heart of learning from the nursing humanities. This being stated, there is little empirical evidence to support the educational effectiveness of using the humanities (Polson and Farmer 2002), so in conclusion it is useful to consider the limited evidence available.

ACTIVITY 4.10

(a) Make a list of books, films, poems, etc. that moved you or where you learnt something about illness or disease or being human. Make the list as diverse as you like. Next to each item make a brief note of the message that you received from the item. It may be that you might like to revisit some of them in the context of your professional practice.

(b) We all have different learning styles and different ways of enjoying the humanities. Which type of materials do you find are most helpful to you – novels, films, drama, photographs and so on? Modify your list from above in which you place the most enjoyable first.

McKie and Gass (2001) evaluate an applied literary learning module in mental health nursing. They identify how it encourages a deeper understanding of complex issues faced in this field but also how care must be taken as to the place of such approaches within the overall curriculum design. Darbyshire (1995: 215) conducted focus groups with participants from a humanities course in Scotland and writes that 'It would be inappropriate to make extravagant claims about the benefits' but he does present many quotes from participants who express its impact as changing them, widening their horizons and how they now think about the way they are as a person.

Jackson and Sullivan (1999) encouraged midwifery students to explore concepts such as caring, empathy, suffering, motherhood, pain, love, attachment, health and illness in the humanities module. Student evaluation revealed they valued the course and had gained insights to develop understanding of these concepts.

In Sweden, a more quantitative approach was taken to student evaluation. An intervention group studied art to discuss characteristics of good nursing care. A statistical difference with a control group was noted where students in the intervention group proved more 'structured, motivated and emotionally balanced when they expressed the elements most typical of good nursing care' (Wikstrom 2001: 25).

In the UK, Kirklin (2001) cites the Bristol inquiry which accused the medical profession of being arrogant, out of touch and misguided and how medical humanities may provide 'both a way to understand and address' these accusations. Her participants demonstrated they learnt there is always another side to a story; how good intention may be insufficient and how really listening to patients can add colour to a typical history-taking event.

In US medical humanities courses, Charon et al. (1995) draw on student evaluations, post-course interviews, questionnaires and faculty assessors to reach their conclusions. They claim the courses improve students' understanding of patients' experiences, support practitioners when dealing with ethical problems and deepen students' self-knowledge in clinically relevant ways. Students secure a better understanding of compassion, recognize their power as health professionals and broaden their horizons through listening, being attentive, seeing and understanding patients through their stories. However, Charon et al. (1995) admit that longitudinal studies are needed to assess the long-term effects.

ACTIVITY 4.11

In conclusion to this chapter, what is your view of the usefulness of the nursing humanities in exploring meaning about illness and promoting patient-centred practice? Write down a few points and discuss them with your learning/tutorial group.

4.6 Conclusion

This chapter has identified the role and influence of the 'nursing humanities' (Darbyshire 1995: 212) as a vehicle to understand multiple meanings of experiences in illness. A range of materials can influence our learning about being human as we engage with accounts of illness and suffering. Reflecting on their meanings offers us opportunities to strengthen our personal and aesthetic knowledge and personal theories (see Chapters 1 and 3). This can positively contribute to our professional judgement in practice and enhance our sensitivity to appreciating needs of patients and their families. Our own journeys through this learning process should be ongoing. There is always a new story to be told whatever the medium of expression. Our motivation should be to listen, to remain open to new possibilities, to reflect, to learn and to enhance our own interpretation and understandings so we not only know more but know better to practise as the people we engage with would have us do.

SELF-EVALUATION

And, finally, your chance to revise what you have learnt from this chapter

1. How would you describe the art and science of nursing?

2. What is the claimed significance of the humanities in nurse education?

3. What materials from the humanities have had an impact on you and why and how did they influence your care practice?

4. What materials would you most recommend to a colleague to discover to influence their practice?

5. What evidence is there to assist in making a decision as to whether the humanities in nursing education promote patient-centred care?

References

Aggleton, P. and Chalmers, H. (2000) *Nursing Models and Nursing Practice.* Palgrave Macmillan, Basingstoke.

Atkins, S. and Murphy, C. (1993) Reflection: A review of the literature. *Journal of Advanced Nursing* 18(8): 1188–1192.

Bauby, J.-D. (1997) *The Diving Bell and the Butterfly.* Fourth Estate, London.

Bishop, A.H. and Scudder, J.R. (1991) *Nursing. The Practice of Caring.* National League for Nursing Press, New York.

Bleicher, J. (1980) *Contemporary Hermeneutics.* Routledge and Kegan Paul, London.

Boykin, A. and Schoenhofer, S.O. (2001) *Nursing as Caring. A Model for Transforming Practice.* National League for Nursing Press, New York.

Bury, M. (1982) Chronic illness as biographical disruption. *Sociology of Health and Illness* 4: 167–182.

Carper, B.A. (1978) Fundamental patterns of knowing in nursing. *Advances in Nursing Science* 1(1): 113–123.

Carson, R.A. (1994) Teaching ethics in the context of the nursing humanities. *Journal of Medical Ethics* 20: 235–238.

Charmaz, K. (1983) Loss of self: A fundamental form of suffering in the chronically ill. *Sociology of Health and Illness* 5: 168–195.

Charon, R., Trautmann, B.J., Connelly, J.E., Hawkins, A.H., Hunter, K.M., Jones, A.H., Montello, M., and Poirer, S. (1995) Literature and medicine: Contributions to medical practices. *Annals* 122: 618–619.

Clark, E. (1992) Psychological perspectives. In: Robinson, K. and Vaughan, B. (eds). *Knowledge for Nursing Practice.* Butterworth-Heinemann, Oxford.

Darbyshire, P. (1994) Understanding Caring through arts and humanities: A medical/nursing humanities approach to promoting alternative experiences of thinking and learning. *Journal of Advanced Nursing* 19: 856–863.

Darbyshire, P. (1995) Lessons from the literature: Caring, interpretation and dialogue. *Journal of Nursing Education* 34(5): 211–216.

Diamond, J. (1998) *'C' because Cowards Get Cancer too... '* Vermilin, London.

Driscoll, J. (1994) Reflective practice for practise. *Senior Nurse* 13(7): 47–50.

Fawcett, J. (1984) The metaparadigm of nursing: Present status and future refinemeuts. *Image* 16(3): 84–89.

Fitzpatrick, R., Hinton, J., Newman, S., Scambles, G., and Thompson, J. (1984) *The Experience of Illness.* Tavistock Publications, London.

Glaser, B.G. and Strauss, A.L. (1968) *A Time for Dying.* Aldine, Chicago.

Gogel, E.L. (1987) Medicine as interpretation: The uses of literary metaphors and methods. *Journal of Medicine and Philosophy* 12: 205–217.

Hargrave, M.P. (1985) New horizons: literary studies in the nursing course. *Australian Journal of Advanced Nursing* 3(1): 39–44.

Hodges, H., Keeley, A., and Grier, E. (2001) Masterworks of art and chronic illness experiences in the elderly. *Journal of Advanced Nursing* 36(3): 389–398.

Illich, I. (1976) *Medical Nemesis: The Expropriation of Health.* Calder and Boyars, London.

Jackson, D. and Sullivan, J.R. (1999) Integrating the creative arts into a midwifery curriculum: A teaching innovation report. *Nurse Education Today* 19(7): 527–532.

Kirklin, D. (2001) Humanities in medical training and education. *Clinical Medicine* 1(1): 25–27.

Kitson, A. (1993) *The Art and Science of Nursing.* Chapman and Hall, London.

Kleinman, A. (1988) *The Illness Narratives.* Basic Books, USA.

Lewis, C.S. (1961) *A Grief Observed.* Faber and Faber, London.

Madjar, I. and Walton, J.A. (1999) *Nursing and the Experience of Illness.* Routledge, London.

Mason, T. and Whitehead, E. (2003) *Thinking Nursing.* Open University Press, Berkshire.

McAdams, D.P. (1993) *The Stories We Live By.* Guildford Press, New York.

McCrum, R. (1998) *My Year Off.* Picador, London.

McKie, A. and Gass, J.P. (2001) Understanding mental health through selected literature sources: An evaluation. *Nurse Education Today* April 21(3): 201–208.

Morse, J.M. and Johnson, J.L. (1991) *The Illness Experience.* Sage Publications, London.

Moyle, W., Barnard, A., and Turner, C. (1995) The humanities and nursing: Using popular literature as a means of understanding human experience. *Journal of Advanced Nursing* 21: 960–964.

Neudert, C., Wasner, M., and Borasio, G.D. (2004) Individual quality of life is not correlated with health-related quality of life or physical function in patients with amyotrophic lateral sclerosis. *Journal of Palliative Medicine* 7(4): 551–557.

Orem, D. (1980) *Nursing: Concepts of Practice* (Second edition) McGraw-Hill, New York.

Parker, D. (1997) Nursing art and science: Literature and debate. In: Marks-Maran, D. and Rose, P. (eds). *Reconstructing Nursing: Beyond Art and Science.* Balliere Tindall, London.

Parse, R.R. (1998) *The Human Becoming School of Thought.* Sage, London.

Parsons, T. (1951) *The Social System.* Free Press, Chicago.

Paterson, J.G. and Zderad, L.T. (1976) *Humanistic Nursing.* Wiley, New York.

Peltzer, D. (2002) *My Story: A Child Called It: The Lost Boy: A Man Called Dave.* Orion, London.

Picardie, R. (1998) *Before I Say Goodbye.* Penguin, London.

Polson, R.G. and Farmer, E.S. (2002) Integrating the humanities in the education of health professionals: Implications for search and revival of information. *Nurse Education in Practice* 2(1): 49–54.

Potter, D. (1994) *Seeing the Blossom.* Faber and Faber, London.

Roach, S.M. (1992) *The Human Act of Caring.* Canadian Hospital Association Press, Ottawa, Ontario.

Robb, A.J.P. and Murray, R. (1999) Medical humanities in nursing: Thought provoking? *Journal of Advanced Nursing* 17(10): 1182–1187.

Robinson, K. (1992) Sociological perspectives. In: Robinson, K. and Vaughan, B. (eds). *Knowledge for Nursing Practice*. Butterworth-Heinemann, Oxford.

Rolfe, G. (1988) *Expanding Nursing Knowledge*. Butterworth Heinemann, Oxford.

Roy, C.C. (1976) *Introduction to Nursing: An Adaptation Model*. Prentice Hall, Eaglewood Cliffs.

Royal College of Nursing (RCN) (2002) *Defining Nursing*. RCN, London.

Schön, D. (1987) *The Reflective Practitioner*. Jossey-Bass, London.

Small, N. and Rhodes, P. (2000) *Too Ill to Talk?* Routledge, London.

Stewart, I. (1929) The science and art of nursing. *Nursing Education Bulletin* 2(1): 1–4 (Editional).

Styron, W. (1991) *Darkness Invisible: A Memoir of Madness*. Jonathon Cape, London.

Throw, M. and Murray, R. (1991) Medical humanities in physiotherapy. *Physiotherapy* 77(11): 733–736.

Watson, J. (1988) *Nursing: Human Science and Human Care. A Theory of Nursing*. National League for Nursing Press, New York.

Wikstrom, B. (2001) Works of art: A complement to theoretical knowledge when teaching nursing care. *Journal of Clinical Nursing* 10(1): 25–32.

Ethics and Health Care

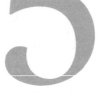

Peter Savage

LEARNING OUTCOMES

This chapter should enable you to

- Explore the distinction between morals and ethics in health care.

- Critically review different approaches to ethical issues in health care.

- Consider the practical application of the different approaches to ethics in health care situations.

- Reflect on the implications of morals and ethics on your professional practice and judgements.

5.1 Introduction

Professionalism in nursing cannot exist without an understanding of ethics to support ethical practice and decision making. The aim of this chapter is to present you with an overview of ethical theories and approaches that are frequently applied to or discussed within health care. Throughout the chapter a number of activities will be presented to encourage you to both explore and apply the theories to practice. These activities include a reflection on your personal views on assisted suicide, banning cigarettes in public places, rationing of health care resources, forced treatments and the character traits of caring. The chapter will begin by defining and then exploring the meaning of the words 'ethics' and 'moral'. This will be followed by an exploration of two theories, utilitarianism and duty-based ethics, that use a deductive approach to ethical justification and decision making. There will then be an exploration of Beauchamp and Childress' (2001) principlism that uses a reflective approach to ethical justification and decision making. Two other theories, virtue ethics and ethics of care, that use an inductive approach to ethical justification and decision making will then be presented. Finally, it will be suggested that a common ground between and including the various theories might exist in terms of a health care ethics. However, as yet such a theory is poorly explained and explored.

5.2 Morals and ethics

The study of ethics stands, as the title of David Seedhouse's (1998) famous book claims, at 'the heart of health care'. However, this may seem odd because some writers, for example Johnstone (1999: 1), have noted that our world view is 'increasingly characterised by moral indiscernability, ambiguity, uncertainty, controversy and perplexity'. One explanation for this is that the value base of health care is somehow divorced from the value base of the society in which health care is practised. However this is such an unlikely development that it may simply be the case that what is required is to disentangle the meanings and significances of the words 'ethics' and 'morals'.

The Oxford English Dictionary (Simpson 2004) definition of 'moral' includes 'a person's lifestyle or self-conduct (especially in sexual matters) considered with regard to morality; a set of personal standards relating to right and wrong conduct.' This definition suggests that morals are to do with personal standards or values. Hence, in a pluralist society that emphasises personal freedom and autonomy, morals and morality acquire a consumerist quality of being more or less what an individual wants. This is then consistent with the quote from Johnstone (1999: 1), concerning 'moral indiscernability, ambiguity, uncertainty, controversy and perplexity'. Thus it is common to find people, even within the same family, holding radically differing views of what constitutes right and wrong on issues such as termination of pregnancy, end-of-life decisions, state funding of health care such as stem-cell research and many others.

However, there remains a requirement to explain why the same types of issues should be at the heart of health care. In order to do so, it is worth noting that the word 'ethics' rather than 'moral' is used in health care. Although these two words are frequently used interchangeably, they can be defined in different ways. The word 'ethics' is derived from the Greek word *ethikos* meaning custom or habit, while 'moral' is derived from the Latin word *moralitas* that originally had the same meaning. The Oxford English Dictionary (Simpson 2004) definition of ethics includes '[t]he rules of conduct recognized in certain associations or departments of human life'.

This definition suggests that ethics are rules, conducts and perhaps values prescribed by a group. All health care professions publish such rules, and examples of such can be found in the Nursing and Midwifery Council's (NMC 2004) Code of Professional Conduct, Standards for Conduct, Performance and Ethics, and the Australian Nursing and Midwifery Council's (ANMC) Code of Professional Conduct for Nurses in Australia. Additionally, many health professions publish what amount to joint position papers on major health issues, for example the British Medical Association's (1999, 2001 update) paper 'Withholding and withdrawing life prolonging medical treatments; guidance for decision making'. Beauchamp and Childress (2001: 7) raise the concern that many such codes of conduct, when scrutinized by moral theory or other sources, may fail to be 'comprehensive, coherent, and plausible', and may be merely self-protective for the professions. The increasing intrusion and power of the law in health care decisions is an example of how professional codes may indeed fail when subjected to close scrutiny. Melia's (2004: 61) begins to explore this matter in relation to decisions concerning what is in the best interest of patients facing death or suffering from chronic debilitating disease. A recent and tragic example of this is the Terri Schiavo case in Florida when the initial decision of health staff to stop feeding Mrs Schiavo and thus allow her death was referred to a higher court by the legislature (a short review of this case is provided by Bhattacharya 2005).

ACTIVITY 5.1

Consider for a moment what your personal views are on the topic of end-of-life decisions. For instance, should a person suffering from an incurable chronic condition such as carcinoma of the bronchi or dementia, who has indicated that they wish to die, be assisted towards their death? Now consider the ethical position of your profession on this topic? A useful paper to read on this is 'Withholding and withdrawing life prolonging medical treatments' (BMA 2001).

5.3 Ethics

It is difficult to obtain a full understanding of the word 'ethics' and there are many ways to disentangle its meaning. One way is to consider ethics as *normative*. By this is meant the identification and justification of the norms of conduct. One way, and a traditional way, to do this is by a process of deductive reasoning.

Here a general theory or principle (or set of principles) is applied to a particular case and the 'right' decision or course of action is determined by a process of deducting from the general theory to the particular case. Utilitarianism and deontology (duty-based) are examples of deductive approaches to ethics (both these approaches will be discussed later in this chapter). Such approaches rely, largely, on something like a scientific approach to ethical decision making in that a principle or duty is applied to particular cases in an abstract, detached and impartial manner.

Reasoning can, of course, be inductive, that is from the bottom up. Thus, justifications or judgements are made in particular cases and from these *norms* can be generalized from the particulars. Sometimes cases are held to be of special import and are termed 'paradigm' cases. The Tony Bland tragedy is an example of a paradigm case. Tony Bland was left in a persistent vegetative state following injuries sustained at the Hillsborough football stadium disaster in 1989. The House of Lords ruling in 1993 permitted the withdrawal of tube feeding and Tony Bland died nine days following the withdrawal of the feeding tube (Melia 2004: 77–78). Virtue ethics and ethics of care generally belong to this approach to ethical reasoning (these approaches will be discussed later in this chapter). These inductive approaches to ethical decision making tend to recognize or even emphasize the particulars of the case in hand and even the individuals concerned with the case.

Beauchamp and Childress (2001) reject both deductive and inductive approaches to health care ethics in favour of, what they term, 'coherence theory'. This is based on John Rawls' (1971) philosophical method called *reflective equilibrium* in which our *considered judgements* (our core moral beliefs) are tested by reflection on our perceptions in particular cases and against moral principles and postulates. The aim is a reflective equilibrium which, Beauchamp and Childress (2001: 399) state, 'is more a process than a finished product; and moral problems . . . should be considered projects in need of continual adjustment by reflective equilibrium'. Beauchamp and Childress (2001) recognize that *considered judgements* require a source and this is, they argue (see Beauchamp and Childress 2001: Chapter 1 and pp. 401–408), in common morality and further that their four principles capture the authority of common morality. Beauchamp and Childress' (2001) four principles will be discussed later in this chapter.

ACTIVITY 5.2

From the viewpoint of a non-smoker, consider the public health issue that cigarettes should be banned from all work places, including public bars. How can you justify this decision and what moral principle, duties or rights apply?

Consider the same issue but imagine that you smoke cigarettes. Are there any differences in your views and if so why and is it possible to overcome any inconsistencies?

5.4 Utilitarianism

Utilitarianism is a type of consequentialism, which asserts that actions are determined right or wrong, good or bad by their consequences. Classical utilitarianism is usually associated with two UK philosophers: Jeremy Bentham (1748–1832) and John Stuart Mill (1806–1873) (see reference to Ryan 1987). Bentham's initial exposition on the principle of utility, 'to promote the greatest happiness for the greatest number, where the happiness of each counts equally' is appealing in its simplicity and its equality. However, from the start it was criticized on a number of fronts, for example its apparent egoism and the real problem presented by a concept like 'happiness'. Indeed, it is more common today to replace the word 'happiness' with 'preference' or even 'welfare'. In this way, utilitarianism is concerned with maximizing the preferences or values of the people concerned.

Additionally, as the principle of utility appeals to the 'greatest number', then it may be open to the charge of justifying neglect or even abuse of individuals if that neglect/abuse serves the interests of most in a society. For example, Beauchamp and Childress' (2001: 209–212) discussion on Quality Adjusted Life Years (QALYs) states, '[t]he problem is that [it] attaches utility only to selected outcomes while neglecting values such as how care is provided . . . and how it is distributed'.

An interesting and famous example of this took place in the late 1980s and early 1990s when the Health Services Commission of the American State of Oregon produced a list of health services to be provided by the state for people on Medicaid (the public health system). Items on the list were ranked according to utility determined by clinical effectiveness and social value (i.e., the preferences of the concerned people gathered by feedback from community meetings). One result of this resource allocation was that funds where allocated to antenatal care (affecting large numbers of women) but not to 'expensive' transplant surgery (affecting a small number of people). This was a rational and democratic approach to health care rationing based on the utility of the ranked items. However, as a result those requiring life-prolonging transplant surgery were left, in the American tradition, to seek charity or other fund-raising activities to pay for their surgery. One such Oregon citizen, seven-year-old Coby Howard who suffered from leukaemia, died whilst raising funds (see Benjamin and Curtis 1992: 99–201 for a review of the Oregon policy and the Coby Howard case).

It is possible to accept the principle of utility, however stated, to determine all ethical decisions. That is, when deciding a course of action we can be guided to produce that which we predict will promote the greatest values/preferred outcomes for the greatest number of people concerned. This is known as act utilitarianism. This can be opposed to rule utilitarianism in which actions are guided by a rule(s) that is deemed to promote the greatest values/preferred outcomes. For example, a rule that maintaining confidentiality of patients/clients will, in the end, promote the greatest value for the greatest number may be applied even if it seems that in a particular case, breaching confidentiality would produce the preferred outcome.

ACTIVITY 5.3

Imagine you have the opportunity to decide five but only five items on which health care resources will be targeted, for example breast cancer screening, antenatal care, or family therapy for mentally ill children. Make a list of your preferences.

Compare your list of preferred health care items with those of a friend or colleague. Which items do you think will most likely get resources and why?

5.5 Duty based ethics (deontology)

The word 'deontology' is derived from two Greek words, *deon* meaning duty and *logos* meaning discourse. Duty-based ethics are old indeed but the version that is most commonly discussed in health care ethics is that associated with the German philosopher Immanuel Kant (1724–1804) (see reference to Paton 1964). For Kant, morality is founded on 'reason' and the ultimate end of reason is 'good will'. In opposition to utilitarianism, reason is autonomous of an individual's desires or preferences (thus unconditional). A law/maxim/duty formulated by reason is thus applicable to all rational beings (thus universalisable) and can be considered a universal law/maxim/duty because its end is 'good will', which is something all rational beings 'must do' (thus imperative). When presented with a conflict between practical considerations and duties, duties must, from this Kantian perspective, take priority (they are categorical). In duty ethics, all duties fulfil the three conditions of being unconditional, universalisable and imperative.

It is possible then to understand how Kant formulated the 'categorical imperative', one formulation of which states, '[a]ct as if the maxim of your action were to become through your will a universal law of nature' (Paton 1964: 89). Thus, once our duties are known to us then we must, in all cases, act on those duties. Additionally, because duties are universal, that is apply to all other rational beings, we must treat all such beings in a manner that respects them as rational beings. Therefore we must '[a]ct in such a way that you always treat humanity, whether in your own person or in the person of any other, never simply as a means, but always at the same time as an end' (Paton 1964: 96).

Kant's influence on contemporary health care ethics is beyond question. Philosophers such as John Rawls (1971) emphasize the Kantian concepts of autonomy and individual worth. Additionally, codes of professional conduct (e.g. NMC 2004, ANMC 2003) are essentially deontological codes that state the duties of the professional, for instance 'you must: protect and support the health of individual patients and clients' (NMC 2004, clause 1.2). Also, research codes that demand informed consent from participants demonstrate the reciprocity principle of treating others as ends, never as means to an end (see, for example, Beauchamp and Childress 2001: 348–355 for a review and evaluation of Kant and Kantian influence on contemporary health care ethics).

There are some problems when attempting both to know and to fulfil our duties. For instance, sometimes duties can conflict. It can be argued that such instances merely demonstrate the incorrect identification of duties, that is, one of the so-called duties is not a duty at all. Nonetheless, the duty to promote a patient's best interest may conflict with the duty to respect the same patient's autonomous wishes concerning treatments. There does not appear to be an oblivious way to resolve this type of dilemma within Kantian-type duty-based ethics.

ACTIVITY 5.4

The NMC (2004) Code of Professional Conduct states that you have a duty to respect the autonomy of patients and clients and also you have a duty to act in the best interest of patients and clients. Imagine you are caring for a patient, who clearly refuses the treatment you believe would benefit them. How would each of the duties, respect for autonomy and acting in the patient's best interest, direct the care you deliver to the patient? Also, how would you resolve any contradictions in the ways that the two duties may direct your care?

5.6 Principlism

The previous discussion focused on deductive ethical approaches. Beauchamp and Childress' 'principlism', certainly in the latest (2001) edition, claims to be a reflective approach to health care ethics. This seems to mean that the 'principles' in principlism can be applied in a soft manner, that is, with sensitivity to the particulars of the case. Implied then is a criticism that the previous methods discussed in this chapter are too abstract, impartial and detached in the application of their principle or duties to cases. As Beauchamp and Childress (2001: 397) state, '[p]rinciples need to be made specific for cases, and case analysis needs illumination from general principles'.

Beauchamp and Childress (2001: 12) present four principles which, they claim, 'express the general values underlying rules in the common morality . . . [and that] These principles can then function as guidelines for professional ethics'. The principles of biomedical ethics are intended to act as guides to action and decision making. Two of the four principles, nonmaleficence and beneficence, 'have played a central role in medical ethics' (Beauchamp and Childress 2001: 12). Indeed, both principles are alluded to in the original code of medical conduct, the fifteenth century BC Hippocratic Oath (Urdang and Swallow 1983: 512). Of the two other principles, justice is an ancient topic within ethical debate though only recently within health care debates. Respect for autonomy owes much to the writings of Kant (see Paton 1964), although Kant's conception of autonomy is founded on the rational principle that autonomous choice is a choice of reason alone uninfluenced by personal desires or preferences.

Beauchamp and Childress' concept of autonomy was, until the 2001 edition, criticized as too individualistic, too libertarian. They respond directly to these criticisms in their current edition, '[w]e aim to construct a conception of autonomy that is not excessively individualistic... not excessively focused on reason... and not unduly legalistic' (Beauchamp and Childress 2001: 57). So autonomy is something like 'at a minimum, self-rule that is free from controlling interference by others and from limitations, such as inadequate understanding, that prevent meaningful choice' (Beauchamp and Childress 2001: 58). Thus autonomy is about self-rule (as the word itself means) but this is limited by the particulars of events that may render some choices to be merely apparent autonomous choices. An example may be that a person's choices are influenced by illicit drugs, medication, disease processes or just the plain influence of another person. For example, the case in which people who have been physically or sexually abused sometimes hide the true nature of their abuse or abuser. However, in such instances respect for autonomy involves not only 'acknowledging decision-making rights [but] enabling persons to act autonomously' (Beauchamp and Childress 2001: 63).

Nonmaleficence (from the Latin *malum* meaning evil and *male* meaning ill), which literally means 'refuse evil', may be the oldest principle of medicine (*Primum non nocere* – first do no harm). Within a health care context, Johnstone (1999: 89) describes nonmaleficence as a 'justification for condemning any act which unjustly injures a person or causes them to suffer an otherwise avoidable harm'. For example, if a patient suffers an infection from a bacteria like methicillin (or multidrug)-resistant *Staphylococcus aureus* (MRSA) because health care workers fail to take simple universal precautions such as properly washing their hands, then that would be a breach of the principle of nonmaleficence.

Beneficence is derived from the Latin words *bene* meaning good and *facere* meaning to do, thus literally to do good. Beauchamp and Childress (2001: 167–173) review the philosophical debate on whether a general obligation to be beneficent exists, that is whether as citizens we have an obligation to do good to or for other citizens. Nonetheless, it is clear that the nature of the relationship between health professionals and their patients/clients establishes an obligation of beneficence. This obligation is frequently referred to as a duty of care. However, a duty of care is clearly also influenced by other principles.

ACTIVITY 5.5

Imagine you have a friend who smokes cigarettes. The friend suffers no ill effects from his or her smoking and when advised to stop, states, 'no harm will come to me and anyway, we all have to die of something'.

Knowing fully well that your friend probably will suffer the ill-effects of smoking, do you think you have a duty (a duty of care) to positively assist your friend to stop smoking and if so, how much assistance should you give and what form should it take?

To offer an example of beneficence, imagine a patient suffering from dementia, in a confused and distressed state asks you to help them 'go home'. Simply returning the patient to a chair in a day room may indeed ensure no harm or danger comes to the patient and this would be an instance of nonmaleficence. However, beneficence guides health professionals to 'do good'. Doing good (acting beneficently) in this instance may require spending time to explore with the patient the nature of their distress and attempting to relieve that distress and confusion. It is not the case that beneficence is a more 'active' principle than nonmaleficence, it is not. Rather it is the case that beneficence demands an orientation to do good and not merely to avoid or prevent harm.

Justice is the most difficult and elusive of the four principles. It is beyond the scope of this chapter to review the literature on this principle; however, Beauchamp and Childress (2001: 225–272) provide a useful review. One conception of justice is termed 'distributive justice'. This concerns, for instance, the just distribution of benefits such as state-funded health care. All such distribution must conform, at least, to Aristotle's formal principle of justice that 'equals should be treated equally and unequals unequally in proportion to their inequalities' (Beauchamp and Childress 2001: 227). Beauchamp and Childress (2001: 234) apply the formal principle of justice through an interpretation of John Rawls' (1971) 'justice as fairness'. In doing this, they claim that state-funded health care means that health care resources and burdens (e.g. taxation) should be distributed equally but in a manner that accounts for inevitable or pre-existing inequalities or in a manner that works for the advantage of all. To argue their case, they claim that health care is needed to ensure what Rawls (1971) terms a 'basic good' (for individuals and society). That is, health care 'is needed to achieve, maintain, or restore adequate or "species-typical" levels of functioning' (Beauchamp and Childress 2001: 234). However, only those aspects of health care that achieve (or are likely to achieve this) have a priority. Thus, emergency care or treatments for acute phases of illness or perhaps preventative health measures/education may be included in state-funded health care but purely cosmetic surgery or artificial fertilization treatments may not be included. Thus they conclude, 'each member of society, irrespective of wealth or position, would have equal access to an adequate, although not maximum, level of health care' (Beauchamp and Childress 2001: 234). As duties may conflict when applied to particular cases, so too may principles guide us in contradictory directions when applied to particular cases.

ACTIVITY 5.6

Beauchamp and Childress (2001: 20) present the scenario, merely to demonstrate a point, that there should be mandatory testing for human immunodeficiency virus (HIV). How would each of the four principles of principlism direct the actions of health care workers involved in this public health issue? For a review of this issue, see Beauchamp and Childress (2001: 15–23).

5.7 Virtue ethics

The next two approaches to ethics, virtue ethics and ethics of care, differ from the above in that they are inductive approaches. Virtue ethics is perhaps most associated, in the ancient world, with Aristotle (384–322 BC) (see reference to Warrington 1963). However, with the rise of 'rationalism' in most aspects of our lives, including ethics, since the European enlightenment of the eighteenth century, virtue ethics has been somewhat neglected. Since the middle of the twentieth century, virtue ethics has made a comeback, in part at least with dissatisfaction with the 'narrow, abstract, impersonal and at times oversimplified approach of traditional theories' (Johnstone 1999: 103). Pellegrino (1995: 254) states, '[v]irtue is the most ancient, durable and ubiquitous concept in the history of ethical theory'. Virtue ethics focuses on the character of the moral agent rather than on abstract principles. It does so by claiming certain traits of character, the virtues, are in themselves morally valuable. Virtues are, according to Pellegrino (1995: 268), 'a trait or character that disposes its possessor habitually to excellence of intent and performance with respect to the *telos* [end] specific to a human activity'. There are a number of ways to 'list' those traits that constitute the virtues, for instance Beauchamp and Childress (2001: 32–38) list compassion, discernment, integrity and conscientiousness. One way of listing the virtues, familiar to many nurses, is Roach's 5 C's of caring, that is compassion, competence, conscience, concern and commitment (see also Chapters 4 and 6). Roach (1987) suggests that these traits are essential components of caring. The habitual operation of these traits, the virtues, constitutes a virtuous or 'good' person. According to Pellegrino, within virtue ethics the virtuous person is 'the person upon whom one can rely habitually to be good and to do the good under all circumstances' (1995: 254).

Virtue ethics holds out the somewhat intuitive approach that some people just are 'good' people and they can be relied upon to do the 'right' thing. Applied to nursing, some nurses are 'good' nurses and are the nurses we would want to care for us or our loved ones if we or they required nursing care. One problem with virtue ethics is that the virtues, whichever list we use, are hard to define and hard to operationalize. That virtue ethicists claim the good person/nurse is the person who habitually does the right thing can seem at best unhelpful and at worst mere deception to the rationalists who advocate deductive approaches to ethics. Nonetheless, virtue ethics can be compatible with the traditional theories, as Beauchamp and Childress (2001: 51) state, '[i]deals transcend obligations and rights, and many virtues dispose persons to act in accordance with principles and rules as well as ideals'.

Further, as noted by Melia (2004: 23), there appears to be a link between virtue ethics and nursing in that virtue ethics emphasizes competency or excellence in performance while nursing has moved towards competency-based training, that is emphasizing excellence in performance. Additionally, virtue ethics links with another approach to ethics that emphasizes the moral agent as part of a relationship and that approach is nursing ethics.

	ACTIVITY 5.7

Remember a time when you or a loved one needed care. Consider the 5 C's of caring, that is compassion, competence, conscience, concern and commitment (Roach 1987), and then describe how each one was demonstrated in the care received by you or your loved? Was it the case that some nurses or other health professionals where better at delivering care and if so, did they more than any other, exhibit the 5 C's of caring?

5.8 Nursing ethics

Melia (2004: 25) states that an '[e]thics of care links to virtue ethics as it focuses on the activities of caring and therefore on the patient–professional relationship and so on the moral agent'. The emphasis in caring ethics is on the motives of any action or decision, how the person performs those actions and on whether the 'actions promote or thwart positive relationships' (Beauchamp and Childress 2001: 370). From a caring ethics perspective, a morally good action promotes the relationships of all involved. Tschudin (1994: 13) describes this as 'social solidarity [in which the] community of people concerned will have gained' by attending to and empathizing with the experiences and emotions of those involved, including the person taking the decision, for example the health care professional.

As with virtue ethics, and for much the same reasons, caring ethicists usually want to reject the abstract, detached and impartial application of principles, duties, obligations or rights and indeed the project of building and testing of ethical theory. Not only does caring ethics focus on the particulars of each case but also, by emphasizing the relationships of those involved, encourages partiality especially towards those 'we care about most and [are] closest to us' (Beauchamp and Childress 2001: 371). This clearly has an intuitive appeal because our moral experiences do suggest that we have a richer commitment to those closest to us and towards whom we care about or love. This is a commitment that deductive ethical approaches tend to ignore in their appeal to impartiality in ethical decision making.

The language of caring ethics is anathematic to many traditionalists such as deontologists or utilitarians. Equally, caring ethicists reject the language of the 'traditionalist'. It is as if they speak in different voices. Indeed, ethics of care developed from the work of an American psychologist, Carol Gilligan (1982). Gilligan's research into the ways that men and women decide ethically suggested that men tended to see morality in terms of rights and justice (hence an ethic of justice), woman tended to see it in terms of empathic associations with and responsibility towards others (hence an ethic of care). It was as if they spoke, as Gilligan's book was titled, *In a different voice*.

Gilligan (1982) avoids attributing the two modes of ethical thinking to mere gender differences. Rather, it is the different psycho-social development (usually) experienced by the two genders that results in the two modes of relationships. The relationship mode of men is towards impartiality, detachment and the ordering of rights. The relationship mode of women tends towards responsiveness, care, prevention of harm and is modelled on the parent–child relationship.

Caring ethics appeals, in particular, to nursing in part because it tends to emphasise those qualities that nurses often appeal to themselves, for example care, compassion, empathy, responsiveness to need and relationships. Additionally, caring ethics recognizes and encourages discussion and decision making that includes those involved with the patient, for example family members. Further, caring ethics presents nursing with an alternative voice to traditional approaches in the debates within health care ethics. Despite Gilligan's (1982) avoidance of genderism, caring ethics became associated with nursing and thus women, as a voice in opposition to the supposedly male world of biomedical ethics.

There are, of course, a number of criticisms of caring ethics (which are reviewed in Beauchamp and Childress 2001: 374–375). Perhaps one of the most serious of these criticisms is the danger of partiality in ethical decision making. For example, one of your relatives or a colleague or a patient you like is admitted to your ward. It does not seem unreasonable to offer them a single room rather than a bed in a 6-bedded bay. Indeed, caring ethics may well encourage this because if allows partiality towards those closest to us. However, this may result in another patient, perhaps one more susceptible to acquired infections such as MRSA, being placed in a more compromising position in a 6-bedded bay. Yet, this is precisely the situation that the more impartial ethical approaches will avoid. Additionally, it is difficult to see just where caring ethicists will draw the line when it comes to those 'closest' to us. This could be interpreted to mean we give ethical priority to those most like us in terms of gender, sexuality, nationality or race and clearly this would be condemned by all the impartialist approaches to ethics.

Tschudin (1994: 9) attempts to overcome this problem, in a model of caring ethics adapted from Niebuhr (1963), when stating that while the 'right' response is not 'based on a theory of duty or achieving goals . . . This does not mean that either duty or the search for good consequences is not considered, indeed it is, as are also all the other ethical guidelines'. Nonetheless, attempts to water down the particularism of caring ethics by appeal to rights, ends and duties is just that, a watering down of the thrust and core of caring ethics.

ACTIVITY 5.8

Consider a patient you have nursed, one with whom you have no particular or special relationship. Now, consider a particular activity you have performed with or for that patient, for example assisting to wash, eat or mobilize.

Now, consider assisting a patient with the same activities but this time imagine the patient is someone with whom you do have a special or particular relationship (a friend, relative or someone similar to your gender, nationality or race).

Are you likely, consciously or unconsciously, to care for the patient who is special to you in a different way to the manner in which you care for the patient who is not special to you? If so, is there a justification for doing so?

5.9 The practice of health care ethics – making sense of the different approaches

Clearly there are a number of differences between the traditional approaches to ethics that rely on the detached, impartial and deductive application of principles, duties or rights and the inductive approaches that focus on character traits, emotional relationships and the particulars of each case. These differences can be emphasized and when this happens there is little common ground for discussion or understanding. This point is demonstrated by the apparent schism between biomedical ethics (doctors, men) and caring ethics (nursing, women). Additionally, within the traditional approaches it is possible for ethical theorists to take a purist approach to the application of their principles or their duties and again this results in little common ground. However, such adherence to theory is probably of little use to practitioners dealing with the always complicated and often messy world of health care ethics.

For some time, a number of writers have attempted to identify and encourage a common ground (Tschudin 1994, Beauchamp and Childress 2001, Melia 2004). This can be criticized as an intellectual muddle, a point identified many years ago by May (1980). Nonetheless this project does seem to fit with much that is real in health care ethics. That is practitioners are, usually, people of good character who do exhibit the traits of caring yet are also directed by theoretical disciplines, one of which is ethical theory. As Melia (2004: 130) states, 'medical ethics and nursing ethics might be better played out as health care ethics' that places patient care at the centre of the project.

The point is that the real issues of practical health care ethics are perhaps best considered in the whole, with practitioners drawing on the many and at times contradictory disciplines that inform health care. Beauchamp and Childress (2001) present a way to progress through the campus of ethics with their application of reflective equilibrium. The problem then is to decide on a starting point on a continuum. Should we start with principles, duties or rights and then allow these to be adapted or bent by the particulars and relationships of each case? This seems to be the position adopted by Beauchamp and Childress (2001). Or, should we begin with the particulars and relationships of each case and allow our moral percepts to be adapted or bent by the knowledge of principles, duties or rights? This seems to be the position adopted by Tschudin (1994). At present, it is not clear that there is a clearly worked out, what Melia (2004) terms, 'health care ethics'.

5.10 Conclusion

This chapter has explored the meanings of and the difference between the words 'ethics' and 'moral'. The chapter then explored approaches to ethical decision making and justification by reviewing two deductive approaches to ethics in health care: the two approaches were utilitarianism and duty-based ethics. Prior to reviewing two inductive approaches to ethical justification and decision making, virtue ethics and ethics of care, the chapter reviewed principlism. Beauchamp and Childress' (2001) principlism was presented as a reflective approach to ethical decision making and justification. Finally, the chapter presented the possibility of an integration of the various approaches to ethics, what may be termed 'heath care ethics' although it was recognized that such an approach has, at yet, to be fully explained and explored.

=========================== **SELF-EVALUATION** ===========================

And, finally, your chance to revise what you have learnt from this chapter

- How would you define the word 'moral'?

- What are your moral views on the topic of medically assisted suicide?

- How would you define the word 'ethics'?

- What is the NMC's views on the topic of medically assisted suicide?

- Describe what you understand by the word 'utilitarianism'?

- Describe a health care situation in which utilitarianism was used to justify an intervention?

- Describe what you understand by the term 'duty-based ethics'?

- Describe a health care situation in which duty-based ethics was used to justify an intervention?

- List the four principles of principlism?

- Describe a health care situation in which one or more of the principles were used to justify an intervention?

- Describe what you understand by the term 'virtue ethics' and list the characteristics that may be considered the virtues of caring?

- Describe what you understand by the term 'ethics of care'?

- Describe a health care situation in which an ethics of care and virtue ethics were used to justify an intervention?

References

Australian Nursing and Midwifery Council (ANMC) (2003) *Code of Professional Conduct for Nurses in Australia*. ANMC, Dickson ACT.

Beauchamp, T.L. and Childress, J.F. (2001) *Principles of Biomedical Ethics*. Oxford University Press, Oxford.

Benjamin, M. and Curtis, J. (1992) *Ethics in Nursing*. Oxford University Press, New York.

Bhattacharya, S. (2005) *Terri Schiavo Dies as Politics and Medicine Collide*. New Scientist [Online] 01 April 2005 http://www.newscientist.com/article.ns?id=dn7222

British Medical Association (1999, 2001 update) *Withholding and Withdrawing Life-Prolonging Medical Treatments*. BMA Books, London.

Gilligan, C. (1982) *In a Different Voice*. Harvard University Press, Cambridge.

Johnstone, M.-J. (1999) *Bioethics: A Nursing Perspective.* Harcourt Saunders, Sydney.

May, W. (1980) Professional ethics: Setting, terrain and teachers. In: Callahan, D. and Bok, S. (eds) *Ethics Teaching in Higher Education.* Plenum, New York.

Melia, K. (2004) *Health Care Ethics.* Sage, London.

Niebuhr, H.R. (1963) *The Responsible Self.* Harper and Row, New York.

Nursing and Midwifery Council (NMC) (2004) *Code of Professional Conduct: Standards for Conduct, Performance and Ethics.* NMC, London.

Paton, H.J. (1964) *Immanuel Kant – Groundwork of the Metaphysic of Morals.* Harper Torchbooks, New York.

Pellegrino, E. (1995) Toward a virtue-based normative ethics for the health professionals. *Kennedy Institute of Ethics Journal* 5(3): 253–277.

Rawls, J. (1971) *A Theory of Justice.* Harvard University Press, Cambridge.

Roach, M.S. (1987) *The Human Act of Caring.* Canadian Hospital Association, Ottawa.

Ryan, A. (1987) *Utilitarianism and Other Essays – Jeremy Bentham and John Stuart Mill.* Penguin Classics, London.

Seedhouse, D. (1998) *Ethics: The Heart of Health Care.* John Wiley, Chichester.

Simpson, J. (2004) *Oxford English Dictionary.* Oxford University Press, Oxford. [Online] 11 October 2004, http://www.dictionary.oed.com

Tschudin, V. (1994) *Deciding Ethically – A Practical Approach to Nursing Challenges.* Bailliere Tindall, London.

Urdang, L. and Swallow, H.H. (1983) *Mosby's Medical and Nursing Dictionary.* CV Mosby, St Louis.

Warrington, J. (1963) *Aristotle's Ethics.* Dent, London.

📖 Suggested reading

On utilitarianism

Singer, P. (1993) *Practical Ethics.* Cambridge University Press, Cambridge.
A useful and popular book that reviews a number of major ethical issues, including termination of pregnancy and euthanasia.

On duty-based ethics

Odenberg, D.S. (2000) *Moral Theory – A Non-Consequentialist Approach.* Blackwell, Oxford.

Odenberg, D.S. (2000) *Applied Ethics – A Non-Consequentialist Approach.* Blackwell, Oxford.
The first book is a presentation of duty-based moral theory and the accompanying book applies the theory to a range of major ethical issues including termination of pregnancy and euthanasia.

On virtue ethics

MacIntyre, A. (1999) *Dependent Rational Animals – Why Human Beings Need the Virtues.* Duckworth, London.
MacIntyre is one of the foremost writers on this subject and this book presents a general view of the theory of virtue ethic.

On ethics of care

Noddings, N. (1986) *Caring – A Feminine Approach to Ethics and Moral Education.* University of California Press, Los Angeles.
This is an important book in the history of caring ethics and also in explaining caring ethics.

Tschudin, V. (2003) *Approaches to Ethics – Nursing beyond Boundaries.* Butterworth-Heinemann, Edinburgh.
A very good collection of essay on ethics of care although it may appear a little complicated for some readers.

General texts

Beauchamp, T.L. and Childress, J.F. (2001) *Principles of Biomedical Ethics.* Oxford University Press, Oxford.

Although the authors clearly argue for principlism in health care ethics, they also provide excellent reviews of most of the topics likely to be debated within ethics. Some readers may find this a rather difficult book to read and it is often best to see at a resource for each topic rather than attempt to read it from cover to cover.

Johnstone, M.-J. (1999) *Bioethics: A Nursing Perspective.* Harcourt Saunders, Sydney.

An excellent textbook that reviews most of the theories and topics in health care ethics.

Kuhse, H. and Singer, P. (1998) *A Companion to Bioethics.* Blackwell, Oxford.

A comprehensive textbook on a range of health care-related topics.

Holland, S. (2004) *Introducing Nursing Ethics – Themes in Theory and Practice.* APS, Salisbury.

A good introductory text to the subject of ethics in nursing.

Rumbold, G. (1999) *Ethics in Nursing.* Baillière Tindall, London.

An easy-to-read introduction to this subject.

Santa Clara University web site http://www.scu.edu/ethics/practicing/decision/approach.html

An easy-to-follow website that provides a range of information on health care ethics.

Caring for the 'Whole Person': Spiritual Aspects of Care

Pauline Turner

CONTENTS

- Components of whole person care

- Definitions of spirituality and spiritual care

- Personhood, relationships and spirituality

- Case study illustrating the spiritual dimensions of caring

- Assessing spiritual care needs

- Spiritual health and distress

- Self-awareness and exploration of own spirituality

LEARNING OUTCOMES

This chapter should enable you to

- Discuss how an understanding of the different dimensions of a person's life may enable you to provide better care

- Describe 'whole person care'

- Discuss definitions of spirituality and spiritual care

- Discuss how relationships form an essential part of spirituality

- Explore ways in which health care professionals can facilitate spiritual care

- Reflect on the development of your own spirituality.

6.1 Introduction

Many people enter health and social care because they want to 'care for people'. They enjoy the interaction with others and often want to be part of a team which helps restore health and function to people who are experiencing ill health. Yet when a person becomes ill, health professionals are not just engaged in fixing the 'part that has gone wrong'. Whether they openly acknowledge it or not, they are drawn into interaction with the 'whole person' – whoever that person might be – and this may involve engaging with many different aspects of a person, sometimes in a way that they had not envisaged. It will often involve seeing the person in the context of their social environment, taking into account their emotional and psychological state, and planning for their physical needs. It should also take into account the spiritual dimension of what 'makes them tick' or who they are at the core of their being. This is particularly important in certain settings, such as chronic illness and palliative care. The aim of this chapter, therefore, is to help you as nurses and health care professionals better understand what constitutes whole person care and how you might address the spiritual needs of patients and clients.

6.2 What do we mean when we talk about 'caring for the whole person'?

Caring for the whole person will involve consideration of the physical, psychological, social and spiritual components of a person's life. The difficulty about talking about it in this way is that people do not present with these separate components and cannot be viewed as such. Each person is a 'whole' and is more than the sum of their individual parts. If my big toe hurts, I, the person who has the toe on the end of her foot, hurt! Health care has often focused on the bits of the body that have gone 'wrong' but there has always been a recognition that we are more than just our 'bodies'. Well over 2000 years ago the Greek philosopher, Plato, is reputed to have said:

> It is impossible to heal the body without knowing something about the soul, indeed without knowing something about the nature of the whole.
>
> (Cited in Moore 1992: x)

It has been suggested that in modern society we have become so preoccupied with the material, physical world that we have lost touch with our 'souls' – what Moore (1992) describes as the inner life of the self. In other words, there is disconnection between the inner life, or self, which is deep down and invisible, and the external (physical and material) world which everyone sees. When someone becomes ill there is usually a diminution, often only temporary, of the external world and this may result in their 'inner life' becoming more prominent. If we are to care for the 'whole person' we need to recognize how important this is and to explore ways in which all the dimensions of a person's life

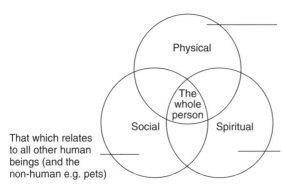

That which relates to all other human beings (and the non-human e.g. pets)

All that pertains to the person's physical make-up, needs and drives, including the brain and whatever mental processes emerge out of cerebral activity, including emotion

That which is 'beyond oneself' and is characterized by openness to the spirit of others, including, but not limited to, other human persons

Figure 6.1 Dimensions of whole person care.
Source: Adapted from Anderson (2003).

can be acknowledged. Anderson (2003) offers us a template of three overlapping spheres (see Figure 6.1) which are useful to consider in the practice of whole person care. As you read Figure 6.1, consider Activity 6.1 and develop your thoughts on this approach.

ACTIVITY 6.1

Take a few moments to think about these dimensions and see if you think any areas are missing. Does the idea of 'inner world' and 'external world' fit these definitions?

Nurses and health care professionals may often find it easier to assess patients' physical, psychological and social needs but there are many dilemmas and challenges involved in assessing spiritual needs (Catterall *et al.* 1998, McSherry and Ross 2002). This may be because education in this area is lacking and tools for assessment are not widely available (Dyson *et al.* 1997, Catterall *et al.* 1998, McSherry and Ross 2002). Yet assessing and providing for people's spiritual, and indeed psychological needs must be considered in a way that is relevant for practice if we are to provide 'whole person' care. How, for example, might the spiritual needs of the 'unpopular' or demanding patient be addressed, or the anxious patient who is facing an uncertain future? What about the patient who has undergone surgery and may be coming to terms with changes in his or her image of themselves? How do we address the spiritual dimension in people who say they have no interest in 'religion' or spirituality? All these questions must be considered if the spiritual dimension of health care is to be understood and implemented in a way that benefits patient outcomes. In Chapter 2, we consider nursing models and how they can guide practice; in this light, work through the suggestions in Activity 6.2.

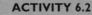

ACTIVITY 6.2

Nursing models represent key concepts for assessing and planning care for patients. Which nursing models do you think promote spirituality as part of the nursing assessment?

Caring for the whole person is especially challenging when someone's life has 'gone wrong' in some capacity and they may find 'wrong' in everything that is done for them. Health care professionals are often called upon to provide the best care for patients and families who may be making unreasonable and even impossible demands upon them. This can put extreme pressures on health carers and give rise to situations described in Activity 6.3.

ACTIVITY 6.3

Half way through her training Sarah (not her real name) said 'Nursing sick people has brought out the worst in me! Sometimes I feel at the end of my tether with people, sometimes just bored. There are patients I positively dislike and I have to summon up all my willpower to care for them. There are times when I wonder if nursing is "right" for me; at other times I know it's what I have always wanted to do and I love it!'

Before reading on think about some of the situations you have been involved in or patients you have cared for where you felt like Sarah – perhaps wondering why you came into health care in the first place. What particular situations/patients make you feel like that?

In the activity outlined above, Sarah, the student nurse, was honest enough to express her feelings about the tough and often demanding job of caring for people like this. But she is at times unable to see how she might view things differently. It is possible that if she were to understand some of the ways in which a person's whole life may be affected by their episode of ill health, it might help her to care more effectively for them (see Chapter 4).

You might be thinking that not every patient or nurse would wish to place as much focus on spiritual care as physical care. However, if a fundamental of care is about promoting an environment which respects and acknowledges the whole person, taking into account a person's spirituality is very important. Indeed spirituality is noted in the International Council of Nurses, Code of Ethics (2000) and the revised Patient's Charter (2001) which puts spirituality firmly in the realm of professional practice (see Activity 6.4).

ACTIVITY 6.4

The International Council of Nurses Code of Ethics for Nurses (ICN 2000: 2) states that 'In providing care, the nurse promotes an environment in which the human rights, values, customs and spiritual beliefs of the individual, family and community are respected.'

The revised Patient's Charter states that 'NHS staff will respect your privacy and dignity. They will be sensitive to and respect your religious, spiritual and cultural needs at all times' (DoH 2001: 29).

Reflect on the ways in which you might adhere to these recommendations. What sorts of approaches and activity would you include?

6.3 So what is spirituality and spiritual care?

One of the challenges in defining spiritual care is to do with its intangible nature. Like 'love' and 'hope' it is a difficult concept to describe fully. Yet it must be defined if we are to make it useful for practice. The word 'spirit' comes from the Latin *spiritus* (Hebrew word *ruach*, Greek *pneuma*) meaning breath, wind – or that which is vital to life. It is essential to and animates the self. It is not about ideas, but lived experience (Robinson *et al.* 2003). It is the vital life source which motivates people (Golberg 1998). This explains why definitions are hard to capture because 'spirit' is embodied within each individual person and has many different forms of expression. It might be described as 'what makes me, me' or 'what makes me tick' (Carroll 2001: 87). Other people have described it as the heart – 'it is only with the heart that one sees rightly, what is essential is invisible to the eyes' – so says the little prince in Antoine de Saint-Exupéry's tale of that name (Saint-Exupéry 2000).

Robinson *et al.* (2003) suggest that the term 'spirit' refers to the sense of life (that which animates), the identity (that which characterizes a person or a group of people) and the qualities of a person or group of people. We can talk about 'a good team spirit'; we talk about people who are 'strong in spirit' as those who are able to face challenges and overcome difficulties; we may have cared for people whose spirit refuses to give up, as well as those who have 'given up'. Illness may deplete a person's resources so being able to nurture and support strength of spirit in people who are ill, or in their caregivers, can be a crucial part of healthcare. The concept of spirituality, therefore, is not just about religious belief but applies to all people and is fundamental to whole person care.

In a study of spiritual care stakeholders from different religious traditions, Wright (2002) found some meaningful definitions of spirituality and spiritual care as follows:

- All people are spiritual beings. The way in which they express their spirituality may be through religious or humanistic beliefs

- Within both religious and humanistic contexts, the concept of 'personhood' (including values and beliefs) and relationships (with self, others and God) figure prominently

- Spirituality goes beyond the here and now – to something beyond ourselves (the transcendent) and has the capacity to search for meaning by addressing the ultimate questions of life and death.

At its simplest, spirituality means making sense of the questions 'Who am I?' and 'What am I?' (Lugton and Kindlen 1999). Within these two simple questions are incorporated wider dimensions to do with culture, belief, the nature of human existence, relationships and identity. A person's sense of self, indeed their sense of meaning and purpose, may be threatened when they become ill (Baldacchino and Draper 2001). A health care professional who has reflected on their own beliefs about meaning and identity will be in a stronger position to affirm and encourage others who are exploring issues of this nature (see Activity 6.5).

ACTIVITY 6.5

What makes you 'you'? Is it to do with something that you 'do', a role you have? Or is it to do with some aspect of who you are, an aspect of your personality? How do you think others see you? Take five minutes and draw or write down all the things that you think people see about you from the outside.

Look at your list and ask yourself 'Does this describe who I am on the inside?'

6.4 What is a person?

Kitwood and Bredin (1992) working in the field of dementia care suggest that having an understanding of personhood is fundamental to developing a theory of dementia care because it is that very sense of having 'lost the person' that creates challenges in caring. Yet the same may be said for the care of people with any condition, not just dementia. Kitwood and Bredin (1992) suggest that personhood refers to the human being in relation to others. The concept of personhood has ethical implications because to be a person is to 'have a certain status, to be worthy of respect'.

There are many different philosophical concepts about the nature of personhood. A view, from a Judeo-Christian perspective, is that people are 'persons' and, by implication worthy of respect, because they are made in the image of God. Others define personhood as consciousness (particularly the capacity to feel pain), to have a sense of self and self-awareness, the ability to reason, to be self-motivated, and to have the capacity to communicate (Warren 1973, cited in Jenkins and Price 1996). Grobstein (1981, cited in Jenkins and Price 1996) suggests that a central criterion of personhood is to be recognized by others, in other words to be accepted in one's own right and thus given attention and concern, love and affection. Similarly, Heyse-Moore (1996) cites an old Zulu saying, 'a person is a person because of people – in other words it is our relationships that make us who we are, whether they be to God, to others, or to ourselves' (Heyse-Moore 1996: 305).

A person's sense of self or identity develops as a social process, first as an infant in relation to its mother or prime carer and then in relation to others as the child matures. Thus personhood emerges in a social context, that is by the presence of others (Kitwood and Bredin 1992: 275). Thus for health care professionals who are seeking to provide care for the 'whole person' having a sense of the relational context in which people grow and develop will help them to care for them and their carers in an appropriate and sensitive way. Relationship with others and with ourselves is also an important part of spirituality.

6.5 Relationships and spirituality

Nolan and Crawford (1997: 291) suggest that spirituality 'has to do with what takes place within, between and beyond people'. It is experienced as relationship on at least four different levels as follows:

1. *How I relate to myself* – the way I see myself. This has to do with a healthy self-esteem and a rejection of pretence in the way I relate to others.

2. *How I relate to others* – defined as a life-long endeavour to appreciate the worth in other people.

3. *How I relate to 'the world'* – this includes social awareness, duties and responsibilities. Personal growth and self-realization are achieved through social interaction.

4. *How I relate to God or the transcendent* – this has to do with that which is 'beyond oneself' and will include belief in God, religious and metaphysical beliefs as well as beliefs about meaning and purpose in life and belief and hope. The devout atheist and the devoutly religious person are equally concerned with describing the world we experience and the purpose of life (Berggren-Thomas and Griggs 1995).

This relational aspect of spirituality makes it impossible to separate spirituality from the psychosocial and physical aspects of being in the world with other people and, if this is so, then every problem we encounter will have a spiritual dimension to it (Carroll 2001) (see Activity 6.6). In the context of health care this means that being able to recognize the spiritual dimension of patients' relationships is an important part of providing whole person care and helping people to develop and grow. It will involve what Cobb and Renshaw (1998: 4) describe as the 'recovery of the patient as a person'.

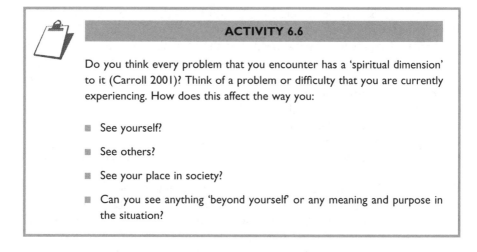

ACTIVITY 6.6

Do you think every problem that you encounter has a 'spiritual dimension' to it (Carroll 2001)? Think of a problem or difficulty that you are currently experiencing. How does this affect the way you:

■ See yourself?

■ See others?

■ See your place in society?

■ Can you see anything 'beyond yourself' or any meaning and purpose in the situation?

6.6 What happens when people become ill?

Earlier in the chapter we referred to Anderson's three overlapping spheres that require health professionals to engage with and to make decisions in: the physical, the social and the spiritual (Anderson 2003). In the case study shown in Box 6.1, it is clear that Roy's physical condition has required intervention by the health care team.

> **BOX 6.1** Case study: Roy
>
> Roy is a 33-year-old father of two young children, being cared for in an acute ward in hospital. His brain tumour has advanced and has affected his ability to swallow. A percutaneous endoscopic gastrostomy tube (PEG) has been inserted through which he is being given regular feeds. He can no longer communicate verbally but he has started to become very agitated every time the feed is commenced. Some of the nurses caring for him are convinced that he no longer wants to be kept alive in this way. His wife, parents and sister are adamant that the feeds should be continued and are becoming hostile to the ward staff – demanding and critical of the care given.

Earlier in the chapter we referred to Anderson's three overlapping spheres that require health professionals to engage with and to make decisions in: the physical, the social and the spiritual (Anderson 2003). In the case study, it is clear that Roy's physical condition has required intervention by the health care team. Anderson (2003) suggests that in this type of scenario the physical sphere often becomes predominant and much of the team's work will revolve around addressing the deficits in the physical domain. The central focus is on maintaining hydration and nutrition and paying attention to Roy's comfort and bodily care. It is clear, too, that his illness is causing profound distress in the family and some of the nurses are beginning to reflect on Roy's distress, associated with his PEG feeds. Clearly, then, the team will need to continue to plan for Roy's care, taking into account his physical needs but they will also need to pay attention to the emotional and social needs of both Roy and his family. If they are to care for him as a 'whole person' they will also need to address the spiritual dimension of who he is and his relationships with others.

It will be important first of all to treat Roy as a person who deserves respect and individualized treatment because he is a unique human being. His distress will need to be alleviated, perhaps by touch, perhaps by the warm presence of another who can 'be there' and attend to his physical needs with care and compassion. In Carroll's study (2001) some of the nurses used massage and played music that was meaningful to the patient as a way of calming and alleviating distress. Conversely, Robinson *et al.* (2003: 20) describe the experience of an acutely ill patient in hospital whose terror, following a nightmare, is unalleviated by the mechanistic approach of the night nurse concerned only with monitoring the machines and supplying drugs. The patient's recovery is significantly aided the next day by the arrival of the hospital chaplain who takes her hand and spends time with her.

Henri Nouwen, a priest, who worked for many years with people with profound learning difficulties wrote about the enormous potential of 'being with' a person:

> Let us not diminish the power of waiting by saying that a life saving relationship cannot develop in an hour. One eye movement or a handshake can replace years of friendship when a man is in agony. Love not only lasts for ever, it needs only a second to come about.
>
> (Robinson *et al.* 2003: 67)

This quality of 'being with' someone in a way that strengthens and comforts is a very important part of spiritual care. Robinson *et al.* (2003) describe this as attending to someone's spirit in a way that becomes central to their recovery. Similarly, Stiles (1990: 245) identified the spiritual dimension of nursing as 'being with' rather than 'doing to'. Campbell (1984) develops the idea of the nurse as being a 'skilled companion'. Greasley *et al.* (2001) identified that users and carers valued the spiritual ethos of nursing care reflected in 'interpersonal values' such as love, care and compassion. These aspects of care are of fundamental importance to patients' well being but may be sidelined and devalued in a system which has emphasized professionalism and the 'mechanics' of care (Greasley *et al.* 2001). In Roy's case it will be the quality of the interpersonal care provided that will help alleviate his distress.

One of the difficulties in recognizing the important contribution of spirituality to a person's well-being may in part result from a Western worldview that tends to value the scientific and more tangible aspects of care above the less visible, interpersonal qualities of 'being' and 'being with' (Turner 1996). Sometimes, nurses and other health professionals are so focused on the 'doing' aspects of their role that they may miss the 'being with' aspect which is so important for people in times of crisis. This is illustrated by an account of a nurse who was reflecting on the death of a patient. The patient's condition had suddenly deteriorated and she was acutely short of breath and distressed. The nurse was sitting at the patient's side, holding her hand. As the patient's fear and distress increased, the nurse's instinctive reaction was to go and see whether a drug had been prescribed which would alleviate this distress. When she returned, the patient was taking her last breaths – alone. On reflection, the nurse wondered why she had thought a drug might be more effective in calming the patient's distress than sitting with her. She was completing a course of study and was very aware of the scientific advances in pain and symptom management. She concluded that the scientific approach emphasized in her studies on symptom management had taken precedence over a more holistic approach (Turner 1996). How would you have acted in this situation? Work through Activity 6.7 to find out.

ACTIVITY 6.7

In the account above, the nurse reflects that in her immediate response to the patient who was dying she gave priority to 'doing for' rather than 'being with' her. Think about your experiences of 'being with' patients. Do you relate to the account above? Have there been times when something (or someone) prevented you from being with a patient. It may have not been what you wanted. What are your thoughts and feelings about that?

I felt _____
I realized _____
I wanted _____

Spiritual care may also involve allowing patients the time and space to work things out or come to terms with their illness. Carroll (2001) describes a story about a dying patient who was argumentative and difficult to nurse. One day he tells one of the nurses:

> I know you lot think I am just lying here sleeping but I am not. I have had a lot of discussions with God, and at long last I realise that he is here for me and does care about me. I am going to talk to him about you lot when I get there. I am ready to go now.
>
> (Carroll 2001: 93)

The sensitivity of the nurses in allowing the patient to deal with things in his own way, whilst still attending to his physical needs, meant that he was able to reach a sense of resolution and inner peace. Although they may not have been able to understand his spiritual concerns, they were able to provide spiritual care by 'being there' and by not judging him. The spiritual dimension is often, by definition, beyond rational understanding. Things will happen for and in patients that health care professionals will have no ability to comprehend. But continuing to care for patients fosters a sense of hope in them (Carroll 2001) and hope may open the door to changed perspectives.

In Roy's case, it may be that his distress is more to do with the loss of the things that had made his life meaningful and an increasing sense of beginning his final journey which, although others can be alongside him, he will have to make on his own. It is often at the end of life that the spiritual dimension comes into clearer focus. In the opening lines of his discussion paper on 'Spiritual issues at the end of life' Hardwig (2000: 28) writes:

> When I am dying, I am quite sure that the central issues for me will not be whether I am put on a ventilator, whether CPR is attempted when my heart stops, or whether I receive artificial feeding. Although each of these could be important, each will almost certainly be peripheral. Rather, my central concerns will be how to face my death, how to bring my life to a close, and how best to help my family go on without me . . . To [most patients and their families], the end of life is a spiritual crisis.

Whether or not Roy is experiencing a 'spiritual crisis' as described above, it is important that the health care team are able to address his spiritual needs as well as those of his family. Although there may not be assessment tools in use on the ward, an ability to distinguish between spiritual 'health' and spiritual distress is very important. Some indicators of these can be seen in Box 6.2 (Newsham 1998). Anandarajah and Hight (2001) describe spiritual distress as being unable to find sources of meaning, hope, love, peace, comfort, strength and connection in life. There may be conflict between a person's beliefs and the reality of what is happening in their life. This conflict may affect their relationships and one way the team may be able to recognize whether Roy is experiencing spiritual distress is by talking with those who know him best. A good starting place might be to ask his family about the things that are important to him, including his beliefs and sources of strength and what might help to support these. It might be helpful to look at his relationships and the way the family are coping with his deterioration, identifying areas of unmet need. Box 6.2 includes indicators which may give clues about whether a person has unmet need in the spiritual dimension. Having made an assessment, it will then be important to decide who might be the best person or persons to address that need. This may not be primarily a problem-solving exercise but may involve the carer showing concern for the patient and offering companionship (Speck 1998). The spiritual dimension of 'being alongside' patients and their families at this time in their lives cannot be overemphasized.

Catterall *et al.* (1998) suggest that the assessment of a patient's spiritual needs must be free from religious, sectarian or any significant bias. Oates (2004) suggests some areas which might be enquired about in a non-threatening way are as follows:

- Reactions to the illness
- How the person views himself/herself with the illness
- How his/her relationships have been affected
- Where the person gets his/her strength from.

BOX 6.2 Concepts around spiritual health and distress

Identifying spiritual health

- Expressing love for others
- Expressing forgiveness by others and God
- Expressing contentment with life
- Expressing contentment in one's value system
- Asking for realistic information about one's situation
- Expressing hope

Identifying spiritual distress

- Expressing lack of support from others
- Feeling isolated
- Expressing guilt
- Expressing anger with self and others
- No reason to live
- Questions about the meaning of suffering
- Expressing despair
- Suppressing feelings
- Failing to wonder or ask questions
- Listlessness and withdrawal

Source: Adapted from Newsham (1998).

However, patients will need to be offered appropriate ways of expressing their spirituality and for many patients this will involve their religious or faith traditions. It will be important for members of the health care team to ensure that they are informed and educated about what is available within their own practice area and be able to act upon it. In many hospitals, the chaplaincy team will have information about the spiritual resources which can be accessed.

Caring for patients like Roy can be a richly rewarding experience if the multiprofessional team is working well together and people are well supported. Relating meaningfully to patients at the end of their lives can 'open the door to the entrance of one person into another's life without it being an inappropriate "invasion" ' (Anderson 2003: 173).

Caring, not only for patients and their families, but for each other in the health care team, is intrinsically spiritual but it needs to be recognized as such and given support and value. Human need can be insatiable and those who take on the role of caring need support to be able to maintain their own spiritual 'health'. Those who care for others need to balance this with care for themselves (Robinson *et al.* 2003). The work environments in which care is delivered need to reinforce this in ways which promote healthy working. Robinson *et al.* (2003) refer to this as professional and spiritual development and suggest that the work environment should include opportunity for space and quiet, reflection and debriefing and an ethos of acceptance and trust where people can relate in satisfying ways. This latter aspect may be on the government's modernization agenda but it needs enormous commitment to carry through.

Developing self-awareness in the area of spiritual care giving may help people develop professionally. Jones (2004) suggests that self-awareness in the area of spirituality may mean that we find it easier to understand the views of those for whom we care. She goes on to say that our responses to others are affected by our past, our upbringing, our concepts of spirituality, and how we find meaning in our lives.

Being able to look at our own beliefs may make us more able to explore with others without feeling uncomfortable. By examining our own beliefs and attitudes we can begin to feel more comfortable with ourselves and ultimately more comfortable with others.

6.7 Conclusion

In this chapter we have looked at some of the dilemmas and challenges in providing spiritual care, a vital component when thinking about caring for the 'whole person' but one which is often neglected in practice. The spiritual dimensions of care are often those which relate to treating people as 'persons', relationships (with God, ourselves and others), finding meaning in illness and suffering and facing the ultimate questions of life and death. We have seen how 'being with' and 'being alongside' people has enormous potential to aid their recovery or to help them prepare for death.

In the case study outlined, we saw ways in which Roy and his family's spiritual needs could be addressed and the importance of adopting a team approach. Those who work in health care also have spiritual needs and the more they are aware of and comfortable with their own beliefs and values, the more likely they are to enhance the care they give to others. There is still a long way to go before spiritual care is routinely incorporated into assessment of the whole person. After reading this chapter you may wish to consider your own philosophy of care and how the spiritual care of patients might be implemented in practice. You may have become aware of areas that you would like to do further reading and reflection on.

━━━━━━━━━━ **SELF-EVALUATION** ━━━━━━━━━━

?

And, finally, your chance to revise what you have learnt from this chapter

■ Look back at the definitions of spirituality (p. 100). How do you experience and express your own spirituality (and/or religion)? If the term has little meaning for you, why is this?

■ What was the model provided by your family? Were they 'spiritually aware'? How was this expressed?

■ Who or what has helped you in times of crisis?

■ Is it possible to find meaning in suffering? How do you cope with suffering?

■ Are there some beliefs which make you feel uncomfortable? What are they? Why do you feel uncomfortable? Is your family model influential here?

Adapted by permission from Dr Shirley Firth. Original material was part of a teaching session on spiritual care at Southampton University.

References

Anandarajah, M.D. and Hight, E. (2001) Spirituality and medical practice: Using the HOPE questions as a practical tool for spiritual assessment. *American Family Physician* 63(1): 81–89.

Anderson, R. (2003) *Spiritual Caregiving as Secular Sacrament.* Jessica Kingsley, London.

Baldacchino, D. and Draper, P. (2001) Spiritual coping strategies: A review of the nursing research literature. *Journal of Advanced Nursing* 34(6): 833–841.

Berggren-Thomas, P. and Griggs, M.J. (1995) Spirituality in aging: Spiritual need or spiritual journey? *Journal of Gerontological Nursing* 21(3): 5–10.

Campbell, A. (1984) Nursing, nurturing and sexism. In: Campbell, A. (ed.) *Moderated Love: A Theology of Professional Care.* SPCK, London.

Carroll, B. (2001) A phenomenological exploration of the nature of spirituality and spiritual care. *Mortality* 6(1): 81–98.

Catterall, R.A., Cox, M., Greet, B., Sankey, J., and Griffiths, G. (1998) The assessment and audit of spiritual care. *International Journal of Palliative Nursing* 4: 162–168.

Cobb, M. and Renshaw, V. (1998) *The Spiritual Challenge of Health Care.* Churchill Livingstone, London.

Department of Health (DoH) (2001) *Your Guide to the NHS.* Department of Health, London.

Dyson, J., Cobb, M., and Forman, D. (1997) The meaning of spirituality: A literature review. *Journal of Advanced Nursing* 26: 1183–1188.

Golberg, B. (1998) Connection: An exploration of spirituality in nursing care. *Journal of Advanced Nursing* 27: 836–842.

Greasley, P., Chiu, L.F., and Gartland, R.M. (2001) The concept of spiritual care in mental health nursing. *Journal of Advanced Nursing* 33(5): 629–637.

Grobstein, L. (1981) *From Chance to Purpose.* Addison Wesley, London. In: Jenkins, D. and Price, B. (1996) Dementia and personhood: A focus for care? *Journal of Advanced Nursing* 24: 84–90.

Hardwig, J. (2000) Spiritual issues at the end of life. A call for discussion. *Hastings Center Report* 30(2): 28–30.

Heyse-Moore, L.H. (1996) On spiritual pain in the dying. *Mortality* 1(3): 297–315.

ICN (2000) *Code of Ethics for Nurses.* ICN, Geneva.

Jenkins, D. and Price, B. (1996) Dementia and personhood: A focus for care? *Journal of Advanced Nursing* 24: 84–90.

Jones, L. (2004) Practicalities of spiritual assessment. *International Journal of Palliative Nursing* 10(8): 372.

Kitwood, T. and Bredin, A. (1992) Towards a theory of dementia care: Personhood and well being. *Ageing and Society* 12: 269–287.

Lugton, J. and Kindlen, M. (1999) *Palliative Care: The Nursing Role*. Churchill Livingstone, London.

McSherry, W. and Ross, L. (2002) Dilemmas of spiritual assessment: Considerations for nursing practice. *Journal of Advanced Nursing* 38(5): 479–488.

Moore, T. (1992) *Care of the Soul: A Guide for Cultivating Depth and Sacredness in Everyday Life*. Harper Collins, New York.

Newsham, G. (1998) Transcending the physical: Spiritual aspects of pain in patients with HIV and/or cancer. *Journal of Advanced Nursing* 28(6): 1236–1241.

Nolan, P. and Crawford, P. (1997) Spirituality in mental health care. *Journal of Advanced Nursing* 26: 289–294.

Nouwen, H. (1979) *The Wounded Healer*. Image Books, New York.

Oates, L. (2004) Providing spiritual care in end stage cardiac failure. *International Journal of Palliative Nursing* 10(10): 485–490.

Robinson, S., Kendrick, K., and Brown, A. (2003) *Spirituality and the Practice of Healthcare*. Palgrave, Basingstoke.

Saint-Exupéry, de A. (2000) *The Little Prince*. Harcourt Brace, New York.

Speck, P. (1998) Spiritual issues in palliative care. In: Doyle, D., Hanks, G. and Macdonald, N. (eds) (Second edition) *Oxford Textbook of Palliative Medicine*. Oxford University Press, Oxford.

Stiles, M.K. (1990) The shining stranger. Nurse–family spiritual relationships. *Cancer Nursing* 13(4): 235–245.

Turner, P. (1996) Caring more, doing less. *Nursing Times* 92(34): 59–61.

Warren, M. (1973) On the moral and legal status of abortion. *The Monist* 57(1): 43–61. In: Jenkins, D. and Price, B. (1996) Dementia and personhood: A focus for care? *Journal of Advanced Nursing* 24: 84–90.

Wright, M.C. (2002) The essence of spiritual care: A phenomenological enquiry. *Palliative Medicine* 16: 125–132.

Suggested reading

Cobb, M. (2001) *The Dying Soul: Spiritual Care at the End of Life*. Open University Press, Buckingham.

Useful and comprehensive insights on spiritual care but as the title suggests mainly from an end-of-life perspective.

Dom, H. (1999) Spiritual care, need and pain recognition and response. *European Journal of Palliative Care* 6(3): 87–90.

Clearly presented material with practical application.

Henley, A. and Schott, J. (1999) *Culture, Religion and Patient Care in a Multi-Ethnic Society: A Handbook for Professionals*. Age Concern, London.

Very useful for identifying culture and faith beliefs and practices in patient care.

McSherry, W. (2000) *Making Sense of Spirituality in Nursing Practice: An Interactive Approach*. Churchill Livingstone, London.

Clear, practical application of definitions and concepts with case study examples from the perspective of nursing practice.

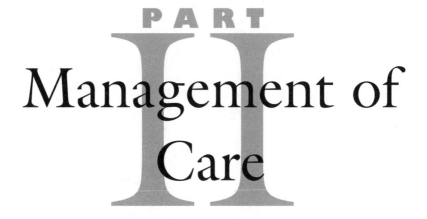

PART

II

Management of Care

The Impact of Health and Social Policy on the Planning and Delivery of Nursing Care

Sue Toward and Sian Maslin-Prothero

LEARNING OUTCOMES

This chapter should enable you to

- Understand the key concepts of policy and health policy

- Describe key themes in health policy in England since 1997

- Discuss the implications of policy changes at national and local levels for nurses, midwives and health visitors, and for the patients they care for

- Reflect on the interplay between politics, policy and power in order to influence decision-makers both at national level and in organizations where nurses, midwives and health visitors work

7.1 Introduction

The aim of this chapter is to explore the impact of policy on practitioners in the United Kingdom (UK). After a brief definition of the key concepts of policy and health policy, some important themes which have shaped health policy since the election of a Labour government in 1997 will be highlighted. It will be argued that these 'themes' are bringing about far-reaching changes not only to the way in which health services are delivered but also to the overall direction of health services in the UK. The impact on practitioners of changes in service delivery and health service priorities will be explored throughout. The chapter concludes with a summary of the key issues and challenges for nurses, midwives and health visitors arising from recent health policy developments.

7.2 Policy, social policy and health policy

There is a widespread perception among practitioners that 'policy' is irrelevant (Robinson 1991, Gough *et al.* 1994). Is it not, after all, something which 'happens' at the level of government and/or in the higher reaches of an organization and which has little impact at practice level? Definitions of policy tend to reflect the important idea that policy has to do with governing (see, for example, Colebatch 2002). Policy is thus concerned with government decisions, actions and activities, all of which have a major impact on a public service such as the National Health Service (NHS). NHS organizations are expected to pursue the overall priorities and specific targets set by government. They will in turn develop local policies, for example in terms of routine practice and procedure, in keeping with the overall framework set by government; for example policy for the appointment of nurse consultants, where the interpretation of the skills and qualifications required of an advanced practitioner differs across the country and organizations. Both managers and practitioners are held increasingly to account for developing their organizations and their practice to reflect government decisions and priorities, such as those set out in the National Service Frameworks (NSFs). It can therefore be argued that the impact of government decisions and actions at practice level has never been greater. In the climate we have described, policy is highly relevant to practitioners.

The NHS is one of the key public services impacting on people's welfare. Hill (2003: 2) suggests that we can think of welfare in terms of the 'basic needs of a society's members', for example for food and shelter, a safe environment, health protection and promotion as well as the treatment and care of the sick, education and training and the care and financial support of those unable to live a fully independent life. Since the 1940s the state has assumed a significant role in providing for the range of welfare needs we have indicated – hence the term 'welfare state'. More generally, policy decisions and actions which influence welfare tend to be referred to as 'social policy' (Masterson 1994).

Health policy can therefore be seen as an area of social policy, but one which needs careful definition. The rest of this chapter will reflect on two distinct meanings of the term 'health policy' and some key themes associated with each. The two meanings are, first, health care policy and, second, policy for health (Hunter 2003).

The central preoccupation of health care policy is with the macro delivery of health care services, for example with how they are structured and financed. As Hunter (2003) puts it, health care policy is concerned with how resources – human, organizational and financial – are used to 'rescue' people who are ill, regardless of the cause(s) of their illness (Hunter 2003: 5). In practice, health care policy tends to be dominated by issues arising from the treatment and care of patients in acute hospital settings. These types of health care facilities or resources lie "downstream" to the causes of illness, for example those arising from the conditions which shape individual and population health (Hunter 2003).

By contrast, policy for health is concerned with improving the health of a whole population, for example by providing the conditions – focusing on non-medical factors – that need to exist in order to keep populations healthy and by tackling various types of health inequality. Policy for health is thus concerned with wider notions of health and its determinants, for example the social, environmental and economic factors affecting health, such as access to education and training, housing, urban deprivation, employment and income levels. These factors are addressed by broader social and economic policy and lie 'upstream' to health services.

When we come to consider important themes which have shaped health policy in recent years, we see the value in seeking to define 'health policy' more rigorously. Most major policy initiatives have been concerned with health services, that is with health care policy. Rather fewer have tackled 'upstream agenda' issues in a coherent 'policy for health' (Baggott 2000, Hunter 2003).

Turning in more detail now to health care policy, we would argue that nine themes emerge very clearly from what has been described as 'relentless, almost hyperactive intervention' in health policy by the Labour government since it came to office in 1997 (Appleby and Coote 2002: 5). These themes – set out below in Box 7.1 – are to be explored mainly in relation to English health care policy. There will, however, be some discussion of the extent to which they have shaped the NHS in Scotland, Wales and Northern Ireland since the introduction of political devolution in 2000. This is further complicated as the Northern Ireland Assembly has been suspended since October 2002; this uncertainty about the political future in Northern Ireland has led to a policy vacuum.

BOX 7.1   The nine themes shaping health policy

  i) Access

  ii) Patient-centred, personalized health services

  iii) Pluralism and diversity

  iv) Primary care-led health services and the shift from hospital to community

  v) Devolution and localism

  vi) Partnership

  vii) Quality and safety

  viii) Modernization

  ix) Marketization.

These nine themes shaping health care policy and their impact on practitioners will now be explored in more depth.

Access

'Access' is an umbrella term for a range of issues about the availability and use of health services, and can be considered as either absolute or relative. Absolute access refers to the overall availability or capacity of health services and also to the timeliness and convenience of services from a patient's perspective. Relative access is concerned more with inequalities in access between different groups. These inequalities may be based on age, sex, ethnicity and culture or a combination of these factors. People are not born with equal health status and it is the stated aim of most governments to reduce the impact of this by seeking to ensure that services are distributed as equitably as possible. Nurses come across people on a daily basis who are excluded or disadvantaged when accessing health care and resources as a result of their personal circumstances, such as their age, mental health status or social circumstances (DoH 2003a,b).

Since 1997 most policy developments to do with access have focused on improving absolute access. Recent significant investment in the NHS – intended to bring UK health expenditure to 9.4 per cent of GDP by 2007/08 to match the European Union average (see Baggott 2004) has been largely used to increase the overall capacity of the NHS so that more patients can be treated and waiting times reduced. Increasingly, stringent targets for waiting times have been set in a succession of policy documents (DoH 2000a, 2002a, 2004a). For example, the 2004 NHS Improvement Plan sets a target of 18 weeks for the whole patient journey from GP referral to hospital treatment (including consultation at hospital level and any diagnostic tests before treatment); this is to be achieved by 2008. Another absolute access target concerns waiting times in primary care, where no patient should have to wait more than 48 hours to see a GP or 24 hours to see a primary care professional (DoH 2000a). Practice nurses have a major role to play in meeting these targets.

Although there is a high degree of consistency in terms of priorities for service improvement between the English NHS Plan (DoH 2000a) and its Welsh equivalent 'Improving Health in Wales' (National Assembly for Wales 2001), overall the Welsh NHS Plan places less emphasis on specific targets and quantified objectives than the English Plan. However, the growing difference in waiting times between Wales and England is leading to the development of more stringent access targets for the Welsh NHS (Ham 2004).

Policies which enable flexible access to services form another important element of the government's strategy to reduce waiting times. Nurse-led initiatives introduced since 1997 include NHS Direct and Walk-in Centres, services which seek to ensure that the NHS delivers more convenient, patient-centred care that meets the needs of modern lifestyles. NHS Direct is a 24-hour nurse-led helpline. Health information and confidential advice are provided on what to do if you or your family are feeling ill, on particular health conditions, local health care services such as doctors, dentists or late night opening pharmacies, and self-help and support organizations. Information and advice can also be accessed electronically from the NHS Direct Online website which is supported by the NHS Direct helpline.

The example of NHS Direct takes us on to our second major theme of patient-centred, personalized health services.

ACTIVITY 7.1

Find out about local service developments which reflect the government's push to improve access to health services.

Are the developments you identify concerned with improving absolute or relative access?

Patient-centred, personalized health services

In the UK, there has been a spate of policy statements since 1997 emphasizing the role of the consumer in determining, shaping and evaluating health services (DoH 1997, 1998a,b, 1999a, 2000b). In future, it is claimed, '. . . the health service will measure itself against the aspirations and experiences of its users' (DoH 1997: 66).

However, there is arguably a growing tension between such statements in policies which were designed to appease and placate users and their represent-atives, and the reality of what has actually been happening. For example, the NHS Plan (DoH 2000a) removed many of the rights given to patients in the Patient's Charter (DoH 1991) and announced the disbanding of Community Health Councils (CHCs), the bodies with a 'watchdog' role in health services and which championed the patients' cause. CHCs were, however, retained in Wales. In England, they have been replaced by a new system of patient and public involvement operating through a number of different groups and mechanisms and which is overseen by the Commission for Public and Patient Involvement in Health (CPPIH). Central to the new system are the Patient Advice and Liaison Services (PALS) providing advice and support in every Trust (DoH 2001d,e). The PALS, which are often run by nurses, offer information and on-the-spot help for patients, their families and carers. The CPPIH also oversees Patients' Forums developed within each community to champion the patient experi-ence and perspective and to host Independent Complaints Advocacy Services (ICAS). The ICAS are independent of the NHS and accessible directly within communities. Not only do they provide support to people who want to complain about NHS services, but they also have the power to look at local NHS provision as part of their wider role in health improvement and in reducing health inequal-ities affecting their area and its inhabitants (DoH 2001d,e). The CPPIH gathers information from these groups and ensures that the relevant organizations are responding to feedback from patients and the public.

With the demise in England of the CHCs and the emergence of these new institutions, the landscape of patient and public involvement has changed consid-erably since 2000. However, there is some evidence that the roles of the new institutions are poorly understood, leading to confusion and even to patient and citizen incomprehension (Health Committee 2003: paragraph 26). The CPPIH and Patients' Forums in particular appear to face an uncertain future.

Since Labour's re-election in 2001, the government has increased the emphasis of putting patients centre stage (Bradshaw and Bradshaw 2004). Improving the overall patient/user experience is identified as one of the four national priority areas in the Department of Health's 2004 'National Standards, Local Action' document (DoH 2004b). The implications of this for practice are wide ranging, although a key idea which comes to the fore is that services should be more patient-centred. Nurses have a key role in ensuring that patients are provided with better information to enable them to be more involved in decisions about their treatment. They can also play a part in facilitating patient choice, whether of alternative treatments or health service providers. At a strategic level, nurses may be involved in obtaining feedback on local health services and in consulting with patients about their future development.

A number of specific policies are designed to improve the 'patient-centredness' of services. For example, by 2008 the Patient Choice initiative (Milburn 2003) will give patients the right to choose to be treated by any health service provider (public, private or voluntary sector), as long as they meet clear NHS standards set by the Healthcare Commission (see Chapter 8) and are able to do so within the national price framework, or tariff, set by the Department of Health (DoH 2004a). Following a decision by the Welsh Assembly government, patients in Wales waiting more than 18 months for an operation are offered the choice of having their treatment at a different hospital (Ham 2004).

A second initiative to make services more 'consumer-focused' is the development of booked appointment systems across the NHS. By the end of 2005, all outpatient appointments and inpatient planned or elective admissions will be pre-booked, for example while the patient is in the GP surgery or outpatient clinic. In effect, this would make waiting lists for hospital appointments and admissions a thing of the past.

ACTIVITY 7.2

Think of an area you have recently worked in. What scope is there for making that service more patient-centred? How could patients be more involved in decisions about their treatment and care, given more choice, or be enabled to provide feedback on services? Try to think of at least two examples.

Pluralism and diversity

One of the consequences of the Patient Choice initiative (Milburn 2003) is that a wider range of health service providers will become involved in providing care and treatment for NHS patients. These providers could be drawn from the ranks of NHS Foundation Trusts in the English NHS (see Devolution and localism theme), from the private and voluntary sectors or indeed from overseas (DoH 2002b,c). Overall the trend, particularly in the English NHS, is for greater diversification or pluralism – more and different types of provider, for example in terms of ownership – in the supply of health services. This trend will be evident not only in the secondary or acute hospital sector. The 2004 NHS Improvement Plan (DoH 2004a) gave a clear indication that the government expects independent (private and voluntary sector) organizations to play a more significant role in primary care provision also. Greater pluralism in the supply of secondary and primary care provision will lead to increasing employment opportunities for nurses in different parts of the non-NHS health sector.

ACTIVITY 7.3

Can you think of any local private or voluntary sector developments such as independent treatments centres (private companies providing elective surgical services to increase NHS capacity: DoH 2002b) which illustrate the trend towards greater diversification in the supply of health services?

Primary care-led health service and shift from hospital to community

In the UK, 86 per cent of all problems brought to the NHS are managed in primary care, with children under 5 and people over 75 averaging as many as seven contacts a year with their GP (Pereira Gray 2003). This, coupled with increased availability and cost-effectiveness of certain medical technologies, goes some way to explaining why, for some years, the overall direction of health care policy has been towards delivering a primary care-led health service. In practice, this implies increasing numbers of services being delivered in primary care or outpatient settings, without the need for hospital admission. In the mental health sector, for example, services have become increasingly community-based with the development of assertive outreach teams, crisis resolution teams and early inter-vention teams (Chisholm and Ford 2004). The growing emphasis on improved management of long term, chronic conditions will further shift the emphasis to primary care (DoH 2004a). These developments, coupled with the European Working Time Directive (EWTD) reducing junior doctors' hours, are opening up an array of opportunities – many of them in community-based settings – for nurses, midwives and health visitors to extend and expand their roles (Chief Nursing Officer [CNO] 2003), for example through community matron posts.

ACTIVITY 7.4

Read through the Chief Nursing Officer's 10 key roles for nurses set out in Chapter 9 of the NHS Plan (DoH 2000a). Find out what new roles for nurses, midwives and health visitors are being developed in primary care settings.

At the macro level, organizational and budgetary arrangements for primary care are being developed to reflect the direction in health care policy we have described. Primary Care Trusts (PCTs), the organizations responsible for the management of primary care services, control over 80 per cent of the NHS budget and a key role in planning and buying, or commissioning, primary and secondary care services on behalf of their patients. In the future, we can expect to see individual general practices being allocated their own budgets and assuming responsibility for what is being termed 'practice-based commissioning' (DoH 2005b). This development is bound to affect referral practice and could create significant differences in the services available to patients both within individual PCTs and between them. It is therefore a controversial aspect of the shift to a primary care-led NHS.

In Scotland, commissioning and purchasing have been integrated; in Wales, the purchaser–provider split has been maintained with an emphasis on partnership; and in Northern Ireland, although health and social care groups have been formed, they are being held back by political uncertainty and there has been difficulty engaging GPs (Smith *et al.* 2004).

Devolution and localism

The growing emphasis on primary care and community-based services highlights our fifth theme, that of devolution and localism. This theme can be explored not only in relation to local services and organizations but also in terms of political devolution. A 'local' interpretation of devolution implicit in the government's stated intention is that responsibility and resources for commissioning and providing health services should increasingly be devolved to local level, for example to PCTs and individual practices. The NHS Plan (DoH 2000a) refers to 'earned autonomy' whereby a decentralization of authority allows managers to manage locally while adhering to standards set by government organizations (such as National Service Frameworks [NSFs]) (DoH 2001a). Staff at the 'front line' will similarly assume increased responsibility for the services they provide. There will be fewer national targets to be achieved and therefore a reduction in central (government-led) bureaucracy and monitoring (DoH 2004a,b). Increasingly local services such as NHS Foundation Trusts in England, although under an obligation to meet national targets and standards like the rest of the NHS, will have greater freedom to decide how they do so. In addition, Foundation Trusts have increased freedom to retain any operating surpluses, for example from land sales, and to borrow money from either public or private lenders (DoH 2002c). They have the freedom to vary staff pay over and above nationally agreed terms and conditions and are more accountable to local people.

At a political level, devolution of power in 2000 to Scotland and Wales has given the Scottish and Welsh governments more control over key policy areas such as health and social care. This has led to some departures in Scotland and Wales from the policy direction set in England. In Scotland, for example, the decision was taken to provide free personal care for older people needing long-term care. The Welsh Assembly government has extended free prescriptions and eye tests, and is committed to phasing out prescription charges all together by 2007 (Ham 2004). Yet there is evidence of some replication of policy such as the Diabetes NSF for Wales that includes new standards for diabetes (National Assembly for Wales 2001). It should be noted, however, that differences in NHS structure in the four UK countries already existed before the introduction of political devolution in 2000.

The devolution and localism theme is a powerful and persuasive one much beloved by politicians from all political parties. There are, however, many examples from health policy which underline how difficult it is in practice for governments to 'let go' of health services in the sense of genuinely devolving responsibility, power and resources to local level. Evidence from Scotland and Wales suggests increased involvement and scrutiny from politicians in the devolved governments. However it is played out, the ever-present tension between central and local level is perhaps best understood in terms of a 'holding on while letting go' dynamic which will most probably continue to characterize the government's relationship with the NHS. As we have stated, policy is, after all, to do with governing and we would not expect a major public service such as the NHS to be unaffected by successive government's values, decisions, activities and actions.

Partnership

As we have seen, policy for health focuses beyond the traditional reach of the NHS to include the wider social, environmental and economic determinants of health. The NHS has limited scope to address these wider determinants of health unless it works in partnership with other agencies which hold more of the 'levers' for tackling the complex and inter-connected problems affecting the health of individuals and communities. Effective partnership arrangements – with local government, the voluntary and private sectors – are considered essential for taking forward policy for health and for improving services. Service provision based on partnership is referred to as integrated care – that is, joined-up working between agencies, in particular local authorities and health organizations, that leads to the effective integration of services for the benefit of service users and carers. This is also described as collaborative, partnership and joint working and the commitment to it is arguably more pronounced in Scotland and Wales than in England (Banks 2002, Wanless and HM Treasury 2002, Integrated Care Network 2003, NHS Scotland 2003a, Scottish Executive 2003). However, partnership has been identified as one of the NHS's 10 core principles (DoH 2000a: see Box 7.2 below) and is intended to be a central feature of health and social care policy; for example, the 2004 'Choosing Health' White Paper (DoH 2004d) identifies working together – to address all the factors that interact to determine health – as one of three core principles of a new approach to public health.

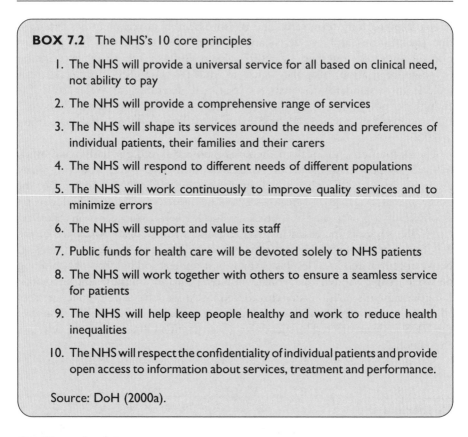

BOX 7.2 The NHS's 10 core principles

1. The NHS will provide a universal service for all based on clinical need, not ability to pay

2. The NHS will provide a comprehensive range of services

3. The NHS will shape its services around the needs and preferences of individual patients, their families and their carers

4. The NHS will respond to different needs of different populations

5. The NHS will work continuously to improve quality services and to minimize errors

6. The NHS will support and value its staff

7. Public funds for health care will be devoted solely to NHS patients

8. The NHS will work together with others to ensure a seamless service for patients

9. The NHS will help keep people healthy and work to reduce health inequalities

10. The NHS will respect the confidentiality of individual patients and provide open access to information about services, treatment and performance.

Source: DoH (2000a).

Quality and safety

The seventh theme, that of quality and safety, evident in health care policy is central to the first health policy White Paper 'The new NHS: modern, dependable' published by the incoming Labour government in 1997 (DoH 1997). This White Paper declared that the NHS would have 'quality at its heart', a challenge taken up in the development of nursing practice and education. The Government's aim is to provide clear, national standards for services supported by consistent evidence-based guidance to raise quality, and to develop a robust system of inspection (see Chapter 8).

All NHS organizations have a system of clinical governance in place to make explicit the responsibility of all NHS staff for quality improvement and safeguarding standards. The Health and Personal Social Services (Quality, Improvement and Regulation) (Northern Ireland) Order 2003 (Department of Health, Social Services and Public Health [DHSSPH] 2003) was laid before the House of Commons. Shortly before its suspension, the Northern Ireland Assembly had begun scrutiny of legislation to establish a clinical and social care governance framework for Northern Ireland. Following suspension, the legislation was re-drafted as an Order in Council. The new legislation brought Northern Ireland in line with arrangements in place elsewhere in the UK specifically, in England and Wales, through the Care Standards Act 2000 and the Health Act 1999, as amended by the National Health Service Reform and Health Care Professions Act (2002); and in Scotland through the Regulation of Care (Scotland) Act 2001.

A senior clinician in every NHS organization is accountable for the proper functioning of clinical governance systems, and chief executives are accountable for clinical standards. A number of key national organizations such as the National Institute for Health and Clinical Excellence (NICE), the Healthcare Commission (formally known as the Commission for Healthcare Audit and Inspection or CHAI), the National Patient Safety Agency (NPSA), and the National Clinical Assessment Authority (NCAA) have been established to help achieve the government's overall aim. Their work, and the wider theme of quality in the NHS, is explored in detail in Chapter 8.

ACTIVITY 7.5

Obtain a copy of the 'National Standards, Local Action' document (DoH 2004b or find it on the Department of Health website www.dh.gov.uk). Look at the seven domains for standard setting; choose two of these and consider the implications the standards set have on nursing, midwifery or health visiting practice.

Alternatively, obtain a copy of a local Trust's clinical governance policy and find out about the clinical governance framework for your current area of practice.

Modernization

The themes we have presented so far suggest the scale of the challenge facing the NHS to develop services which reflect not only the demanding aspirations the government has for health care but also the changing needs and increasing expectations of patients and users. The reform and modernization of services – emphasized in the English, Scottish and Welsh NHS Plans – is considered fundamental to achieving genuine and sustainable improvements. Modernization seeks to transform the way in which services are provided through the redesign of the way people work and of the systems and technologies they use. Nurses and other health care staff will constantly have to adapt to the challenge of working in new ways as modernization transforms service delivery. The NHS Modernization Agency (www.modern.nhs.uk) was set up in April 2001 to support the NHS and its partner organizations in modernizing services. The government now believes that much of what the Modernization Agency set out to do in terms of providing strategic support for the implementation of the NHS Plan (DoH 2000a) has been achieved and therefore proposes to slim down the Agency by 2005 (DoH 2004c).

ACTIVITY 7.6

What examples of modernization have you come across in practice? Find some examples of service redesign and of staff working differently.

Marketization

The final theme we have identified in relation to health care policy is that of marketization. This suggests that a range of market-style disciplines – for example contracting and competition – are increasingly being used to bring about improvements in service quality and efficiency and to enhance patient-centredness and choice. Despite the Labour government's claims that it is opposed to a market in health care, it seems clear that the NHS – particularly in England – is increasingly operating on the basis of competition. For example, PCTs with their key role in commissioning primary and secondary care services on behalf of their patients enter into contracts with a range of health service organizations for the provision of these services. Service providers, whether they are NHS organizations, or based in the private or voluntary sectors, compete to win contracts. The government's intention is that by 2008 providers will be paid on the basis of the volume of work or activity they undertake. The price providers are paid for the work they carry out is to be set at national level, thus removing prices from local negotiation. This means that competition among providers will be based not on price but on a range of other factors, for example on the degree of patient choice, quality, shorter waiting time, volumes of activity and efficiency. Overall, this policy is known as 'payment by results' (DoH 2002a), and there are indications that it could be extended to cover services outside hospital settings, such as primary and community care services. The theme of marketization would thus have a profound impact across the whole spectrum of health care services. Nurses will have a key role in ensuring that the types of factors – including patient choice and quality – fundamental to success in the health care marketplace are reflected in the services they are involved in delivering.

7.3 Policy for health

The challenges arising from health care policy developments in recent years, for example reducing waiting time seem more than sufficient to keep health care professionals and managers fully occupied. And yet increasingly the NHS is being asked to turn its attention to what Hunter (2003) has termed 'policy for health'. In the NHS Improvement Plan (DoH 2004a), the government sets out a vision of an NHS being transformed 'from a sickness service to a health service'. According to this view, waiting will cease to be a major issue, freeing up the NHS to focus on disease prevention and tackling inequalities in health. This could signal increasing emphasis being put on themes which have been evident in UK public health policy since 1997.

For example, a number of policy initiatives have focused on areas of inequality and social exclusion with the aim of improving the health and health care of communities (DoH 1997, 2000a). The first wave of Health Action Zones (HAZs) – partnerships between the NHS, local authorities, community groups and the voluntary and business sectors – were introduced in April 1998. The HAZs reflect the important idea that responsibility for improving health cannot be seen as the exclusive domain of the Department of Health. Issues such as child poverty and inequality have to be tackled across all government departments, agencies and sectors. A total of 26 HAZs were established in England in areas of deprivation and poor health to tackle health inequalities and modernize services through local innovation. The HAZ communities vary significantly in their local characteristics, but they face common problems of ill health and disadvantage. They represent areas in England with some of the highest levels of deprivation and the poorest levels of health; for example in Manchester, Salford and Trafford, four areas identified for priority help include children and young people, people with a mental illness, older people and supporting organization change by engaging communities, front-line staff, the private and public sector and other interested parties in a partnership approach (DoH 1999b). HAZs aim to develop and implement a health strategy that reduces inequalities, and deliver within their areas measurable improvements in public health and health outcomes, and in quality of treatment and care. They aim to increase sustainability by developing contacts with other zones, by disseminating ideas more widely, and by playing a major role in joining up existing initiatives (HazNet 2001). These partnerships are required to be developed across statutory, voluntary and private sectors; for projects to be funded they must be realistic and have a clear purpose, for example improve educational standards in poor areas or reduce unemployment among young black and minority ethnic males. Another initiative is Health Improvement Programmes (HImPs) which aim to focus on the most important needs of the population. These also encourage cross-sectoral working, between the NHS and local authorities. The first examples were launched in April 1999 and they assessed local needs, mapped resources, identified priorities and developed strategies for change. Taken together, HAZs and HImPs provide opportunities for community nurses, with their expertise and knowledge of local social, economic and environmental issues, to lead and contribute (see Box 7.3). For joint working to be successful, the different groups involved need to overcome their historical, cultural and financial boundaries (Arora *et al.* 1999).

BOX 7.3 Case study: Catherine Baraniak

Catherine Baraniak is a primary care nurse in Derby who as a result of the NHS (Primary Care) Act 1997 is the UK's first nurse contract holder of a GP practice – she employs a GP and a team of nurses (Leifer 2005).

This case study provides a positive example of a nurse embracing the new opportunities in community settings. Changes in government policy allow nurses to be entrepreneurial. For example, the Personal Medical Services (PMS) contract offers opportunities for nurses to

- Hold the primary contract in primary care

- Be the first point of diagnostic and therapeutic contact for patients

- Have more responsibility in the planning of primary care

- Occupy both a clinical and a managerial role

- Lead general practice services in areas where there are inadequate numbers of doctors.

In the same year that saw the launch of HImPs, the government also published a strategy for health called 'Saving Lives: Our Healthier Nation' (Secretary of State for Health 1999). This focused mainly on the disease-based areas of cancer, coronary heart disease and stroke, accidents and mental illness and set objectives and targets for reducing the death rate associated with each area. The disease-based approach of 'Saving Lives' was not without its critics, however. Claims were made that it reflected the medical model and paid too little attention to the wider health improvement agenda of supporting communities to stay healthy and tackling the growing health gaps between rich and poor (Hunter 2003).

The NHS Plan (DoH 2000a) contained just one chapter on improving health and reducing health inequalities, suggesting that it was more concerned with health care policy than policy for health. This contrasts with the Welsh and Scottish NHS Plans (National Assembly for Wales 2001, Scottish Executive 2001). Arguably these are more focused on population health improvement and strategies for achieving it – for example multi-sectoral and partnership working – than on health care (Hunter 2003). However, the one overtly 'policy for health' chapter in the English NHS plan did announce a commitment to developing national targets for health inequalities. These were subsequently published in March 2001 (DoH 2001b). In the same month, the Chancellor of the Exchequer commissioned a major review to examine future health trends and the resources required to provide a publicly funded and high quality health service. A key conclusion of the review team was that 'better public health measures could significantly affect the demand for health care' (Wanless 2002 [1.27]: 6). In other words, health promotion and sickness prevention could significantly improve the population's health status and thus result in lower demands for health care as well as improved productivity in the working population. Good health is thus seen as good economics. Yet there are concerns about health inequalities between western, central and eastern parts of the World Health Organisation (WHO) European region and the health of children and adolescents across the European Community (Europa 2003, WHO 2003a,b).

Two years later, in 2004, the Wanless review team published a further report, this time focusing on ill health prevention and wider health determinants. It also explored the cost-effectiveness of action to improve the population's health and reduce health inequalities. The government's response to the second Wanless report and the overall direction of policy for health was set out in a White Paper 'Choosing Health: Making healthier choices easier' published in November 2004 (DoH 2004d). This makes it clear that two major themes will be significant in shaping future policy for health. These are described below.

Health and health gain / health improvement and reducing health inequalities

As already noted, this theme is more explicit in the Welsh and Scottish NHS Plans than in the English equivalent. However, since 2000/01 improving the health of the population has been identified as one of four national priority areas

(DoH 2004b) with a set of national targets to be achieved by 2010. These are broadly concerned with increasing life expectancy by reducing mortality rates from specific diseases or causes (heart disease and stroke, cancer, suicide and undetermined injury), by reducing health inequalities and by tackling some of the underlying determinants of ill health and health inequalities, for example smoking, obesity and the under-18 conception rate.

Policy for health is further developed in the 2004 'Choosing Health' White Paper (DoH 2004d) which sets out a raft of measures – some new, some already underway – aimed at improving health and tackling health inequalities. Overall the emphasis is on the government, communities and the NHS supporting individuals to make 'better' – that is healthier – choices for their health and for the health of their families. For example, the government will legislate to ban smoking in enclosed public places and work places by the end of 2007. The food and advertising industries will face increasing restrictions on the promotion to children of unhealthy foods. The government will work with the food industry to enable the clear, unambiguous labelling of the nutritional content of food. A national campaign targeting those at risk of sexually transmitted infections or unplanned pregnancies will be mounted, and a chlamydia screening programme accelerated to cover all England by 2007. The government has also made a commitment to continue to work to address the wider causes of ill health and inequality in health, for example through policies to tackle social exclusion and childhood poverty.

According to the White Paper 'Choosing Health' (DoH 2004d), the NHS will increasingly become a health improvement and prevention service as it seeks to focus on supporting individuals to make and maintain healthy choices. As the largest staff group in the NHS workforce, nurses will have a very significant role to play across primary care, through hospital care to specialist services in ensuring that the estimated 1.5 million contacts people have with the NHS every day become opportunities for health improvement and promotion. A new National Health Competency Framework will identify the training and support nurses, and other NHS staff, need to develop their understanding and skills in promoting health. In addition, nurses who already work in a health improvement service, for example smoking cessation or nutrition advice, will have the opportunity for additional training and skills development. Health visitors will be responsible for leading specific initiatives such as the Child Health Promotion programme and new roles for school nurses are also envisaged. For example, School nursing services are to be modernized and expanded in order that by 2010 primary and secondary schools will have access to a team led by a qualified school nurse (DoH 2004d).

The examples we have given of specific health improvement measures set out in 'Choosing Health' (DoH 2004d) underline the high priority the government intends to give to this aspect of policy for health. In addition, we also see increasing emphasis being put on improving the support available to people with long-term conditions. It is to this second national priority area (DoH 2004b) that we now turn.

ACTIVITY 7.7

In health policy there is an on-going debate about the respective responsibilities of government, the NHS, practitioners and individuals in improving
health. Read the Executive summary of 'Choosing Health' (DoH 2004d).
Does the White Paper strike the right balance in terms of the expectations
and responsibilities of the groups we have identified?

Long-term/chronic conditions

Chronic conditions have been defined as 'diseases which current medical interventions can only control not cure. The life of a person with chronic disease
is forever altered – there is no return to normal' (DoH 2004e: 3). In the
UK, an estimated 17.5 million people suffer from chronic conditions which
require long-term care and advice over years. The most common such conditions are asthma, dementia, diabetes, hyperlipidaemia and hypertension (Pereira
Gray 2003). A number of risk factors – for example high blood pressure and
cholesterol, obesity, physical inactivity and abuse of alcohol, tobacco and other
substances – are often the precursor to chronic disease. At a global level, the
World Health Organisation (WHO) has identified that 60 per cent of the world
disease burden is attributable to chronic conditions (WHO 2002).

Given the enormous challenge posed by chronic disease at both a national
and a global level, it is perhaps surprising that the health policy agenda – at least
at the domestic level – has traditionally been dominated by the drive to reduce
waiting lists for elective care. Politically the treatment and management of
long-term conditions has tended to be a much lower priority, possibly because
of the numbers of people affected and the subsequent cost implications. In the
changing climate towards chronic disease, however, health professionals face
a formidable challenge. This not only consists of educating and empowering
people to live less dangerously but also to manage their chronic illness more
effectively, ensuring that the best long-term advice and care is made available.
A number of initiatives – for example the Expert Patient Programme (DoH
2001c) and community matrons (DoH 2005a) – are designed to help health
professionals and their patients and carers to rise to the challenge we have
described. For example, the case management role of community matrons will
involve the identification of those whose health is at greatest risk and partnership
working with the patient to tackle the effects of disease and prevent hospital
admission.

The fundamental overhaul of NHS priorities inherent in a shift away from
health care policy (the downstream agenda) to policy for health (the upstream
agenda) will not be without its tensions, nor can it take place in a political
vacuum. Not only will health professionals have to adapt to changed roles and
ways of working but they will also need to grapple with a number of more
general political issues and challenges, and it is to a consideration of these that
we now turn.

7.4 Key issues and challenges for nurse, midwives and health visitors arising from recent health policy developments

The NHS currently employs over 350,000 nurses, and nursing is the largest of the health professions and the biggest staff group in the NHS workforce (DoH 1999a). Nurses utilize significant resources in order to deliver or directly supervise the majority of direct care provided by the NHS. What nurses do and the manner in which they perform their work directly influences quality, costs and the patient's experience. As a result, clinical effectiveness and cost efficiency are significantly affected by the way in which nurses practice and are organized and deployed (DoH 2000a).

In the NHS Plan (DoH 2000a) and Choosing Health (DoH 2004d), the government outlined its commitment to preventing as well as treating ill health and reducing health inequalities. Challenging the current inequitable access to health and health care resources, economic impoverishment and unsafe physical surroundings which threaten the health and well-being of countless people requires an understanding of the nursing contribution not only in terms of service delivery but also in shaping the policy process itself. Nursing and health care are clearly areas for political activity and debate as scarce resources are allocated amongst competing and arguably equally worthy groups and needs; for example health care policy and policy for health could be seen as representing competing causes when it comes to resource allocation. It is essential for nurses to be accepted by the wider policy community and be thinking in a politically informed way if they are to have the issues they are concerned about taken seriously (Hart 2004).

Currently, nurses work in health care systems that still exclude or disadvantage large numbers of people needing care and are frequently confronted by health problems caused by ageism, sexism, racism and the inequitable distribution of resources. Despite explicit commitments to health promotion, nurses tend to focus on patients/clients as individuals and on the minutiae of the nurse–patient relationship rather than the macro socio-political context of health and health care. Nurses can bring about change in health and social policy and arguably this should be seen as an aspect of professional responsibility; in the UK nursing's statutory regulatory body the Nursing and Midwifery Council (NMC) states in the Code of Conduct that: 'As a registered nurse, midwife or health visitor, you must: protect and support the health of individual patients or clients; protect and support the health of the wider community' (NMC 2004: 4). Although there have been some positive role models in the past, such as Florence Nightingale and her contribution to the development of the profession and recognition of the importance of the vital area of infection control, or Chris Hart and his call to nurses to be politically astute, nurses rarely challenge the structures within which they work and do not tend to address fundamental issues such as inequality that may determine health status, permeate health care structures and can constrain nurses' ability to deliver health care, possibly because of the difficulty in presenting a united front.

NHS Chief Executive Sir Nigel Crisp (DoH 2004f) described nursing leadership as 'pivotal' to patient-centred care, leadership and influencing the future. He said nursing leadership was key:

- *In championing better health and services for local people* – nurse leaders should help people contribute to a new vision of health and care

- *Within a reforming NHS* – where clinical standards are more transparent and public confidence hinges on getting the fundamentals of care right

- *Professionally* – ensuring that nursing continues to produce high quality leaders from all parts of the community.

Under the Knowledge and Skills Framework (DoH 2004g), all staff covered by Agenda for Change, whether nurses, health care assistants, porters or cleaners, must show that they can develop and apply the appropriate knowledge and skills, for example to reduce the risks of health care associated infections such as MRSA. The infection control role of nurses is seen as one of the best ways of limiting the spread of infections (DoH 2004f) – through personal development plans staff and managers have an opportunity to identify how to raise standards of cleanliness.

In order to achieve this change in perspective and mode of practice, nurses need to understand health and social policy, the provision of health care and the structures within which that health care is provided. The ability to challenge the marginalization and subordination of the nursing voice in current political debates is dependent on this knowledge. That is, policy cannot be influenced or shaped unless it is recognized and understood (Maslin-Prothero and Masterson 2002).

7.5 Conclusion

In this chapter we have argued that a broad understanding of policy and policy implementation at local and national level is of fundamental importance in order for nurses to influence proactively the health agenda for health gain. In the UK nurses' limited awareness of, and engagement with, the health policy agenda may go some way in explaining nurses' historic invisibility in terms of influencing policy. The ability to understand and challenge the marginalization and subordination of the nursing voice within policy decision-making circles as well as in the face of medicine is dependent upon this knowledge. Such a large and diverse profession as nursing has faced difficulty in achieving a single voice on many political and professional issues, and policy makers and policy analysts have consistently shown their disregard for nurses. As the Chief Nursing Officer has highlighted (DoH 2004f), policy changes that have major implications for nurses, their work and the patients they care for are imposed upon them with little reference to them, their needs or interests; and policy analysts at best pay cursory attention to nurses and their analyses. The boundaries between the different health care disciplines and the nature of the structure and funding of health care are fluid rather than fixed and are historically and socially constructed by the complex interplay of power between different groups. However, analyses of the type modelled in this chapter help policy makers and analysts better understand the contribution of nursing and nurses to health care. Such awareness, we believe, can facilitate the best use of nursing and nurses for social good.

═══════════════ **SELF-EVALUATION** ═══════════════

And, finally, your chance to revise what you have learnt from this chapter

■ Name two policy documents published since 1997 which identify new ways of working in a modernized health service.

■ From your own experience in practice can you identify at least two examples of new roles and/or career developments in health and social care?

■ Since 1997 the relationship between health care professionals and patients has been changing. Based on your reading and experience highlight three changes you have observed.

■ Modernization has endeavored to change the way in which services are provided; both in the way people work and the systems and technologies they use. In light of this, talk to friends, family and colleagues to identify three new models of service delivery at local level that have resulted from NHS modernization.

■ Implementing 'policy for health' requires a response across all government departments, agencies and sectors. This is leading to an increase in multi-agency and interdisciplinary working and learning.

■ Reflect on your own experience and give an example of a multi-agency and interdisciplinary approach to (a) working and (b) learning.

References

Appleby, J. and Coote, A. (2002) *Five Year Health Check. A Review of Government Health Policy 1997–2002*. King's Fund, London.

Arora, S., Davies, A., and Thompson, S. (1999) *Developing Health Improvement Programmes: Lessons from the First Year*. King's Fund, London.

Baggott, R. (2000) *Public Health Policy and Politics*. Palgrave, Basingstoke.

Baggott, R. (2004) *Health and Health Care in Britain* (Third edition). Palgrave Macmillan, Basingstoke.

Banks, P. (2002) *Partnerships under Pressure*. Kings Fund, London.

Bradshaw, P.L. and Bradshaw, G. (2004) *Health Policy for Health Care Professionals*. Sage Publications, London.

Chief Nursing Officer (CNO) (2003) *Rising to the Challenge of the Working Time Directive. The CNO Bulletin*. Department of Health, London. [Online] www.doh.gov.uk/cno/bulletindetail_nov.htm#topnews

Chisholm, A. and Ford, R. (2004) *Transforming Mental Health Care*. Sainsbury Centre for Mental Health, London.

Colebatch, H.K. (2002) *Policy* (Second edition). Open University Press, Maidenhead.

Department of Health (DoH) (1991) *The Patient's Charter.* HMSO, London.

Department of Health (DoH) (1997) *The New NHS: Modern, Dependable.* The Stationery Office, London.

Department of Health (DoH) (1998a) *Our Healthier Nation. A Contract for Health.* The Stationery Office, London.

Department of Health (DoH) (1998b) *Health in Partnership: Patient, Carer and Public Involvement in Health Care Decision Making.* Department of Health, London.

Department of Health (DoH) (1999a) *Making a Difference: Strengthening the Nursing, Midwifery and Health Visiting Contribution to Health and Health care.* Department of Health, London.

Department of Health (DoH) (1999b) Health action zones. In: Department of Health (ed.) *78 Million Pound Trailblazing of Money for Modernisation.* Department of Health, London.

Department of Health (DoH) (2000a) *The NHS Plan. A Plan for Investment. A Plan for Reform.* The Stationery Office, London.

Department of Health (DoH) (2000b) *NHS Research and Development Funding. Consultation Paper: NHS Priorities and Needs.* Department of Health, London.

Department of Health (DoH) (2001a) *Shifting the Balance of Power with the NHS – Securing Delivery.* Department of Health, London.

Department of Health (DoH) (2001b) *Tackling Health Inequalities. Consultation on a Plan for Delivery.* Department of Health, London.

Department of Health (DoH) (2001c) *The Expert Patient: A New Approach to Chronic Disease Management for the 21st Century.* Department of Health, London.

Department of Health (DoH) (2001d) *Involving Patients and the Public in Health Care: Response to the Listening Exercise.* Department of Health, London.

Department of Health (DoH) (2001e) *Shifting the Balance of Power.* Department of Health, London.

Department of Health (DoH) (2002a) *Delivering the NHS Plan: Next Steps for Investment, Next Steps on Reform.* The Stationery Office, London.

Department of Health (DoH) (2002b) *Growing Capacity: A New Role for External Health care Providers in England.* Department of Health, London.

Department of Health (DoH) (2002c) *A Guide to NHS Foundation Trusts.* Department of Health, London.

Department of Health (DoH) (2003a) *Tackling Health Inequality: A Priority for Us All.* Department of Health, London. [Online] 02/07/03 www.doh.gov.uk/healthinequalities/programmeforaction

Department of Health (DoH) (2003b) *On the State of the Public Health.* Department of Health, London. [Online] 03/07/03 www.doh.gov.uk/cmo/annualreport2002

Department of Health (DoH) (2004a) *The NHS Improvement Plan: Putting People at the Heart of Public Services.* The Stationery Office, London.

Department of Health (DoH) (2004b) *National Standards, Local Action. Health and Social Care Standards and Planning Framework 2005/06–2007/08.* Department of Health, London.

Department of Health (DoH) (2004c) *The Future Direction of the NHS Modernisation Agency. Statement on the Future Direction of the NHS Modernisation Agency.* Department of Health, London.

Department of Health (DoH) (2004d) *Choosing Health: Making Healthier Choices Easier.* The Stationery Office, London.

Department of Health (DoH) (2004e) *Chronic Disease Management. A Compendium of Information.* Department of Health, London.

Department of Health (DoH) (2004f) *Chief Nursing Officer's Conference 2004,* Manchester, 3–5 November 2004. Department of Health, London. [Online] (Date) http://www.dh.gov.uk/NewsHome/ConferenceAndEventReports/ConferenceReportsConferenceReportsArticle/fs/en?CONTENT_ID=4097515&chk=mdHshD

Department of Health (DoH) (2004g) *The NHS Knowledge and Skills Framework (NHS KSF) and the Development Review Process.* Department of Health, London.

Department of Health (DoH) (2005a) *Supporting People with Long Term Conditions: Liberating the Talents of Nurses Who Care for People with Long Term Conditions.* Department of Health, London.

Department of Health (DoH) (2005b) *Commissioning a Patient-Led NHS.* Department of Health, London.

Department of Health, Social Services and Public Health (DHSSPH) (2003) *Health and Personal Social Services (Quality, Improvement and Regulation) (Northern Ireland) Order 2003* http://www.ni-executive.gov.uk/press/hss/030108d-hss.htm

Europa (2003) *The Health Status of the European Union. Narrowing the Health Gap 2003* http://www.europa.eu.int/comm/health/ph_information/documents/health_status_en.pdf

Gough, P., Maslin-Prothero, S., and Masterson, A. (1994) *Introduction. Nursing and Social Policy: Care in Context.* Butterworth Heinemann, Oxford.

Ham, C. (2004) *Health Policy in Britain: The Politics and Organisation of the National Health Service.* Palgrave Macmillan, Basingstoke.

Hart, C. (2004) *Nurses and Politics. The Impact of Power and Practice.* Palgrave Macmillan, Basingstoke.

HazNet (2001) *A Fully Interactive Site for Sharing the Experiences of Health Action Zones in Tackling Health Inequalities.* Department of Health, London.

Health Committee (2003) HC697. 7th Report 2002/03 *Patient and Public Involvement.* The Stationery Office, London.

Hill, M. (2003) *Understanding Social Policy* (Seventh Edition). Blackwell, Oxford.

Hunter, D. (2003) *Public Health Policy.* Polity, Oxford.

Integrated Care Network (2003) *About Integrated Care.* Department of Health, London. [Online] 16/06/06 http://www.integratedcarenetwork.gov.uk/themes/integration.php supported by the Care Services Improvement Partnership.

Leifer, S. (2005) Focus primary care: My practice. *Royal College of Nursing Bulletin* 9: 2

Maslin-Prothero, S. and Masterson, A. (2002) Power, politics and nursing in the United Kingdom. *Policy, Politics and Nursing Practice* 3(2): 108–117.

Masterson, A. (1994) What is social policy? In: Gough, P., Maslin-Prothero, S., and Masterson, A. (eds) *Nursing and Social Policy: Care in Context.* Butterworth Heinmann, Oxford.

Milburn, A. (2003) Choice for all. Speech made by the Secretary of State to NHS Chief Executives, 11 February 2003. Department of Health, London.

National Assembly for Wales (2001) *Improving Health in Wales: A Plan for the NHS with its Partners.* National Assembly for Wales, Wales.

NHS Scotland (2003a) *Partnership for Care: Scotland's Health White Paper* http://www.show.scot.nhs.uk/sehd/publications/PartnershipforCareHWP.pdf

Nursing and Midwifery Council (NMC) (2004) *The NMC Code of Professional Conduct: Standards for Conduct, Performance and Ethics.* Nursing and Midwifery Council, London.

Pereira Gray, D. (2003) 2020 vision. *Health Service Journal* 2 October: 18–19.

Robinson, J. (1991) Power, politics and policy analysis in nursing. In: Perry, A. and Jolley, M. (eds) *Nursing: A Knowledge Base for Practice.* Edward Arnold, London.

Scottish Executive (2001) *Our National Health: A Plan for Action, a Plan for Change.* Scottish Executive, Edinburgh.

Scottish Executive (2003) *Community Health Partnerships.* 18 July 2003. http://www.scotland.gov.uk/consultations/health/comhealpart.pdf

Secretary of State for Health (1999) *Saving Lives: Our Healthier Nation.* HMSO, London.

Smith, J., Mays, N., Dixon, J., Goodwin, N., Lewis, R., McClelland, S., McLeod, H., and Wyke, S. (2004) *A Review of the Effectiveness of Primary Led Commissioning and its Place in the NHS.* The Health Foundation, London.

Wanless, D. (2002) *Securing Our Future Health: Taking a Long-term View. Final Report.* HM Treasury, London.

Wanless, D. and HM Treasury (2002) *Working Together: Effective Partnership Working on the Ground.* HM Treasury, London.

Wanless, D. and HM Treasury (2004) *Securing Good Health for the Whole Population. Final Report.* The Stationery Office, London.

World Health Organisation (WHO) (2002) *Innovative Care for Chronic Conditions: Building Blocks for Action.* The World Health Organisation, Geneva. [Online] 03/02/05 http://www.who.int/chronic_conditions/en/icccglobalreport.pdf

World Health Organisation (WHO) (2003a) *Health Systems Confront Poverty.* http://euro.who.int/observatory/toppage

World Health Organisation (WHO) (2003b) *The Health of Children and Adolescents in WHO's European Region.* http://www.who.int/child-adolescent-health/New_Publications/NEWS/doc53.pdf

@ Useful websites

www.dh.gov.uk   Department of Health
www.chai.org.uk   Healthcare Commission
www.modern.nhs.uk   NHS Modernisation Agency

Suggested reading

Baggott, R. (2004) *Health and Healthcare in Britain* (Third edition). Palgrave Macmillan, Basingstoke.
This book is a clearly written text which provides students with an up to date and concise introduction to all aspects of health care in Britain today. It also covers political changes such as the health policies of the UK Government since 1997 and the increasing diversity of the NHS as a result of devolution.

Hill, M. (2003) *Understanding Social Policy* (Seventh edition). Blackwell, Oxford.
This offers a concise history and understanding of social policy in the United Kingdom.

CHAPTER

Quality and Clinical Governance

Rob Carter

LEARNING OUTCOMES

This chapter should enable you to

- Define what is meant by 'quality care'.

- Understand the principles and concepts enshrined within TQM.

- Recognize quality as being a key concept within contemporary health and social care.

- Understand what is meant by 'clinical governance'.

■ Recognize the roles of those organizations who have a quality-monitoring remit.

■ Appreciate your professional responsibilities under the NMC Code of professional conduct

8.1 Introduction

Ever since the inception of the National Health Service (NHS) in July 1948, the objective of achieving quality has been a central feature of organizational life. Its very *raison d'etre* was to improve the standard of health for all the people of the United Kingdom. Labour's first Secretary of State, Aneurin Bevan, announced the Bill to the House of Commons which launched the NHS. He famously set out the principles upon which the NHS was to be established. This was to make the best advice and treatment available to all regardless of a person's level of income, and to provide everybody, no matter where they may live, with the same level of service (Klein 2001).

Although there can be no doubt that the NHS has achieved a great deal in terms of improving the health of the nation, particularly during the early years having made major inroads into defeating serious conditions such as polio and tuberculosis, the issue of whether it is able to provide everyone with the best care has been a subject of considerable debate. This in the main has been due to pressure on resources coupled with increasing expectations by users of the service.

Quality then, as a concept, has been redefined and articulated over the years in order to meet the different and changing expectations of consumers. Just as we all quite rightly expect our individual expectations to be met when we purchase a particular product or service from a business in the high street, in the same vein we demand similar levels of service from those who work in health and social care settings. This presents health care professionals with a serious challenge of how to achieve quality in such a way as to meet the ever changing needs of clients/consumers of services. This chapter and its associated learning activities will help you to understand your role in rising to such a challenge.

8.2 What does quality mean?

Some important thinkers

Deming

Deming (1986) is probably one of the earliest and most notable figures within the quality movement. He developed his ideas whilst assisting Japanese industry to reconstruct and modernize during the post-war era. Tellingly, many of his key ideas which are credited with helping Japan to emerge as a major global economic power were not taken up until much later by the so-called victorious and more traditional industrial nations such as the United States and Britain. Arguably, this gave Japanese companies a stronger competitive edge over their rivals. Deming was able to recognize that constant change was to become an increasingly familiar feature of organizational life and as such organizations providing products or services needed to adapt themselves continuously, in order to meet the changing demands of consumers (Deming 1986). Central to his ideas on how to improve quality was the recognition that it should be an all-embracing concept in which everybody involved has an important contribution to make. This concept has become known as Total Quality Management, which is more familiarly abbreviated as TQM. Although TQM will be explored later in this chapter, it is worth stating here that its central point is that everyone is recognized as being mutually dependent on others within their team and beyond in ensuring a quality product or service is provided.

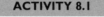

ACTIVITY 8.1

Seven ways of defining care

1. Comfort of patients

2. Proportion of people under care, by gender and age per group

3. Number of people kept out of hospital by good community care

4. Facilities for tests, such as laboratories, X-ray, etc

5. Public health programmes

6. Average mean age of people discharged from hospital

7. Amount of money spent per patient/client

These are different ways in which Deming (1986) describes how the quality of care may be defined. Each of these are, however, open to interpretation, for example under the first point, how do you measure comfort?

What sort of things would you need to consider in qualifying the other six statements?

Juran

Like Deming, Juran (1986) worked on the reconstruction project in post-war Japan. He is credited with providing his own very succinct definition of quality which is merely stated as 'fitness for purpose' (Juran 1986). Simply put, if the item or service, such as a particular drug or level of nursing care, fits the purpose for which it is intended, then it fulfils the requirements of quality. Juran also views the wider benefits to be gained by putting quality at the very top of the agenda, because in doing so it helps to reduce costs and results in improvements in productivity. Valuable time may be saved in rectifying problems, thereby focusing efforts on other areas of activity.

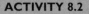

ACTIVITY 8.2

All nurses and other health care professionals recognize the importance of effective hand-washing in preventing the spread of infection. Despite this, poor practice is thought to be a contributory factor in causing high rates of contraction of MRSA in many British hospital settings. Improvements in practice should lead to reductions in transmission of infection, shorter hospital stays and a lower risk of readmission for patients. This leads to better patient outcomes, and beds becoming available more quickly to treat new patients.

Try to identify the potential costs (both financial and human) associated with poor practice here.

8.3 Defining quality

Arriving at a universally agreed and acceptable definition of what quality means is difficult. We tend to have different views of what quality means based on our own understanding and experience. Literature provides us with a variety of definitions such as 'conformance to requirements' (Crosby 1984). Although on one level if the requirements are being met, it might be assumed that quality is being achieved, this particular definition does not appear to take account of the costs that might be involved. Taking this definition at its face value might suggest that the duty to provide everything the customer requires is necessary to ensure quality is achieved regardless of costs. Within a publicly accountable service such as the NHS, there are bound to be limits placed on expenditure, and so in arriving at a workable definition of quality, it is helpful to recognize who the interested parties might be in determining what quality is.

Øvretveit (1992) has identified three different dimensions of health service quality and in doing so has aligned them with their respective interest groups. They are

1. *Client quality* – what patients, clients and carers at an individual or wider population level want and expect from the service.

2. *Professional quality* – does the service meet the required needs as defined by the various professionals and those who make referrals, and are the most appropriate procedures and technology available.

3. *Management quality* – are resources used to their optimum efficiency within the constraints and directives established by those who purchase and commission services on behalf of patients, clients and carers.

From looking at Øvreveit's dimensions, it is possible to identify occasions when there may be conflicts of interest between the three. A clear example of when sometimes conflicts arise might be when there has been a media report on a new area of pioneering medical practice. In 2003 for example, the first successful procedure took place in the United States to give a patient a fully functioning artificial heart. This was widely reported in the media, possibly fuelling demands from patients and patient groups in this country, that a similar procedure should be available on the NHS.

From a professional standpoint, this particular procedure was very much in its infancy. The skills and technology required to carry out such a procedure would need to be acquired, and this could require amongst other things considerable time and training. In addition, the professional viewpoint is likely to be longer term in wanting to establish an evidence base for how successful the procedure might be in terms of patient outcomes.

From a management position, the cost of developing the means whereby such a procedure might be available could be prohibitive. New therapeutic and technological developments, particularly in the field of health care, are notoriously expensive. Managers need to determine whether resources are being used to the best effect.

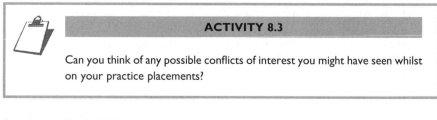

ACTIVITY 8.3

Can you think of any possible conflicts of interest you might have seen whilst on your practice placements?

Another well-established view of providing dimensions against which quality can be assessed is given by Maxwell (1992).

ACTIVITY 8.4

Based on Maxwell (1992) dimensions of quality

1. Access – are services near-by, how long do they have to wait, are there any barriers such as poor car parks, distance to walk?

2. Equity – does the provision of service take account of cultural, racial or social background?

3. Relevance to need – is the overall provision of service a reflection of the needs of the population as a whole?

4. Social acceptability – how sensitively are the services provided in terms of patient dignity, privacy and confidentiality?

5. Efficiency – are services optimally delivered within available resources and how does the cost of the service compare with other providers?

6. Effectiveness – are services the best available in terms of evidence-based care, which can be demonstrated by achieving good patient outcomes?

ACTIVITY 8.4 continued

From your practice placements, can you identify positive and negative examples of these dimensions at work? You could also assess the quality of a service which you or a member of your family has used.

What would you do to improve things?

8.4 Patient-centred care

In response to the report into the failings in children's cardiac surgery at Bristol Royal Infirmary, the Secretary of State has made it clear that patient-centred care needs to be a core feature of everything the NHS does in the twenty-first century (DoH 2001). The importance of patient-centred care has also been emphasized within the government's strategic document, the NHS Plan (DoH 2000). According to Kendall and Lissauer (2003), for high quality patient-centred care to exist, five key characteristics need to be present.

Kendall and Lissauer's (2003) five broad features providing a framework for high quality patient-centred care:

1. *Care should be safe and effective* – there needs to be an emphasis on evidence-based care to ensure it is safe, and that the best health outcomes are achieved for patients.

2. *An emphasis on promoting health and well-being* – there needs to be the dual benefit of treating people for existing conditions, and also preventing further ill health by the promotion of good health practice.

3. *Care should be integrated and seamless* – a holistic approach to care will improve patient outcomes, and should involve the coordination of services within the NHS and between it and other sectors such as social care in both the public and private areas of provision.

4. *Care should be informing and empowering* – health professionals need to give patients high quality information so that they can contribute to and make informed choices about the decisions affecting their care.

5. *Care needs to be timely and convenient* – successive patient surveys reveal that a top priority for patients is that services are timely and responsive to their needs. Inappropriate delays to treatment not only have the effect of possibly worsening patient conditions, but they also add to the costs (Wanless 2002).

ACTIVITY 8.5

After considering the issues which might contribute to a working definition of 'quality' in health and social care, try to come up with your own definition. In a single sentence, produce a definition which should take account of the patient/client, level of care, outcomes and costs/resources.

8.5 Key terms and concepts in 'quality'

Total Quality Management (TQM)

Total Quality Management takes the principles of quality further by suggesting that it should be extended to every part and individual within the organization. In a hospital setting, this means that the TQM philosophy should be driven by the Chief Executive and will be jointly shared and owned by all staff in every department, from ancillary workers (cleaners, porters, etc.) through to senior professionals and managers (consultants, human resource director, etc.). TQM is about prevention of poor practice and so a good deal of effort needs to be invested in the elimination of mistakes. The idea of getting things 'right the first time' is very important in the TQM approach. Writers such as Deming (1986), Crosby (1984) and Oakland (1993) have identified the principles necessary for TQM to be delivered. Coincidentally they all conclude that 14 steps are required, which for our purpose here have been conveniently summarized down to 6 main ones by Henderson (1998).

Requirements for TQM

1. *Commitment and leading by example from senior management* – the case for the primary importance of quality needs to be made at a senior level and regularly emphasized.

2. *Organization-wide commitment to quality* – the emphasis on making quality improvements needs to be shared at an equal level across all parts and departments of the organization, recognizing that there is a mutual interdependency.

3. *Strong emphasis and focus on the customer* – a recognition that the ultimate objectives should be about achieving customer satisfaction.

4. *An approach to working which engenders participation and teamwork* – this means harnessing the enthusiasm of staff in getting them to personally deliver quality care and services.

5. *Quality of suppliers* – this recognizes that the organization, for example hospital, cannot work in isolation and that it is often dependent on external suppliers offering a quality service, for instance food, drug, cleaning suppliers, and so on.

6. *Pursuit of continuous improvement* – this means constantly finding out how good the services are by asking your customers and then acting upon suggestions of how things can be improved.

Zero-defects

Crosby (1984) identified that in pursuit of continuous improvement an approach needs to be followed which aims to eliminate or minimize errors and mistakes. Even though 100 per cent eradication of mistakes is unlikely to be achievable, it should be the ultimate target. This has the dual benefit of ensuring that everyone is focused on achieving excellence, and also that the pursuit of quality is a never-ending continuous process.

To illustrate the strength of the zero-defects approach in confirming that no amount of non-conformance is acceptable (Parsley and Corrigan 1999), the issue of the safe prescribing and administration of drugs can be used. Drug errors can have potentially fatal consequences. Having said this they do still unfortunately occur. When mistakes take place it is important to ensure that particular errors are not repeated in the future. The zero-defects concept quite rightly advocates that the seriousness of this approach in the area of drug errors should be extended to all other aspects of patient and client care.

Example

If five needle-stick injuries occur in a day when overall 500 needle-stick proced-ures are carried out, this represents a safe administration rate of 99 per cent.

Using the zero-defects approach, another way of interpreting this is that over the course of a year 1825 injuries might occur.

ACTIVITY 8.6

Using the zero-defects approach think of some examples of your own when you have witnessed mistakes/errors occurring and try to estimate the consequences of not taking any action.

Quality chains

Quality chains are a useful way of illustrating the TQM approach. It is possible to visually represent the interdependency of different individuals and departments within an organization by constructing a 'quality chain'. The concept of quality chains begins with the premise that each link within a chain may be viewed as an important supplier of a service to the next link, who is in turn a customer to the preceding link. It follows therefore that the customer is also a supplier to the next link. This process continues until the ultimate service to the customer, most likely the patient or relative, is received. Like all chains, they are only as strong as their weakest link. As Morris (1989) points out, quality is required at every link to ensure that the chain is not broken, leading to a failure in service at the end of the chain. The end represents the interface, usually between the organization and the patient. Using this approach, it is possible to interpret customers as being not only external (patients, relatives), but also internal (other members of staff, professionals, departments).

ACTIVITY 8.7

Think of an episode of care involving a referral of a patient by their family doctor to an ENT outpatients clinic at the local district general hospital. Construct a quality chain, indicating the parties involved from the point of referral, to the end of the episode in outpatients. Try to think quite widely, including the effects such things as car-parking, sign-posting, and so on might have on the overall quality of the patient experience. This activity should also demonstrate the complexity of what might seem at first sight a straight-forward process.

8.6 Why is quality important?

As has already been stated, quality has always been an issue of importance within the NHS. Over the past 20 years or so, the requirement to focus on patients as consumers, in much the same way as private service providers view their customers, has gathered pace. The recommendations from the Griffiths Report (DHSS 1983) advocated amongst other things the necessity for the NHS to view patients as customers. The NHS and Community Care Act (1990) pursued the agenda further, with the introduction of a quasi-internal market for health care. This provided for the first time a truly competitive environment in which purchasers of health care could theoretically agree contracts of patient care with a range of providers, based on the joint criteria of cost and quality. Providers of services who were to be heavily dependent upon the success of winning and retaining such contracts would therefore feel incentivized to make improvements in quality.

The recognition that patients were to be seen as consumers was institutionalized by the Patient's Charter (DoH 1991), which set out national rights and service standards that patients could expect (Baggott 2004). These were to mainly include issues around access, such as waiting times, but also consideration and respect, the provision of information, and complaints. The Charter has been revised and expanded to include specific groups such as children and the mentally ill.

The emphasis on quality and the importance of a consumerist approach has been continued under successive Labour governments since 1997. They had been quick to recognize and interpret public dissatisfaction in the NHS as a rationale for furthering consumerism (Baggott 2004). The White Paper 'New NHS: Modern, Dependable' (1997) set out Labour's plans for the NHS. The theme of quality dominates the content of the White Paper, introducing a robust new regime of inspection in health and social care. In addition, it sets out an agenda to tackle inequity in health care provision, and to improve quality in some key target areas of health such as coronary heart disease and strokes, and cancer care.

From a strategic policy viewpoint, we can see why quality is such a prominent feature in contemporary health and social care. It does of course have to translate at the level of delivery. Henderson (1998) provides three compelling reasons as to why quality is important:

1. *Importance to patients* – quality is of benefit because patient requirements are met and outcomes are good. Additionally, a good patient experience should enhance their confidence in the service for the future. This will have the effect of reducing the level of anxiety and stress in patients and relatives.

2. *Importance to staff* – staff in health and social care are motivated by their commitment to provide a good service to their patients and clients. Well organized, resourced, good quality care will lead to greater job satisfaction, positive patient feedback and an enhanced reputation for the department.

3. *Importance for reducing costs* – although there is often a cost associated with providing good quality, poor service invariably leads to a waste of money (Carruthers and Holland 1991). Higher costs may be associated with investigations following complaints, repeating procedures due to lost records, readmissions because of too early discharge, and so on.

8.7 Clinical governance

The focus on quality is central to the government's approach to the management of care (Hewison 2004). Following the Bristol Royal Infirmary Inquiry (Kennedy 2001) and its associated recommendations, the government was compelled to address the issue of quality in ensuring that the tragedies of Bristol could not be repeated elsewhere. Its key proposals which had been set down in 'New NHS: Modern, Dependable' (DoH 1997) were taken forward and substantiated in A First Class Service (DoH 1998). This document proposed that the health care sector should embrace a comprehensive and fully accountable quality assurance framework, to be known as 'clinical governance'.

Quality assurance has been described as the measurement of the actual level of the service provided, together with the efforts to modify when necessary the provision of these services, in the light of the results of the measurement (Williamson 1978). The brief of clinical governance was to go beyond this rather narrow definition of quality assurance, in providing a root and branch framework on quality, consistent with the principles of TQM. Clinical governance is defined as:

> a framework through which NHS organisations are accountable for continuously improving the quality of their services and safeguarding high standards of care by creating an environment in which excellence in clinical care will flourish.
>
> (Scally and Donaldson 1998: 62)

In translating this into something more user-friendly for health care professionals, the Royal Berkshire and Battle Hospitals NHS Trust (2004) define the concept as:

> Clinical governance is about the patients and their carers receiving the right care at the right time by the right person in a safe environment.

The challenge for health service managers is in ensuring that the appropriate strategies are in place for this to occur. One of the major criticisms in the past of the NHS is to do with the high degree of variation in terms of cost and quality of services. This has led to inequity in both the availability and standards of care. In this sense, clinical governance needs to be viewed as an all-embracing concept which should be interpreted broadly as a means of improving the overall quality of care throughout the NHS (Bloor and Maynard 1998). It implies the involvement and cooperation of all health care professionals, support staff and managers.

At a wider level, the clinical governance strategy requires the development of new evidence-based guidelines, providing agreed standards of care. Once these have been established and agreed, they are then monitored by a statutory body, the Healthcare Commission. Those who commission health care locally are then able to assess the performance of health professionals, ensuring that they practise the best clinical care which is also cost-effective. Ultimately, the aim is to balance financial probity with clinical quality.

The aim is to move from unacceptable variation to acceptable variation.

McSherry and Pearce (2002) point out that clinical governance is not just about having appropriate systems in place to ensure that mistakes are not made. It is also about instilling the public and health care professionals with a level of confidence, secure in the knowledge that they are in a safe and adequate clinical environment. A First Class Service (1998) suggests that local health care organisations comply with the following nine goals:

1. establishing views of patients
2. validating the quality of data
3. evidence-based practice
4. assessing risk
5. lead responsibilities on clinical governance
6. quality assurance in clinical practice
7. inform staff and patients about quality systems
8. clinical leadership
9. education and training

The seven pillars of clinical governance

The Commission for Health Improvement (CHI) now operates as the Health care Commission carrying out regular reviews of health and social care organizations in both the public and private sectors. Reviews look at clinical governance from the three angles of patient experience, the clinical team and the corporate strategy, which includes the systems and processes used for monitoring and improving services. This is assessed using the seven pillars of the clinical governance framework (CHI 2003).

The following are the seven pillars:

1. *Patient involvement* – how the public, stakeholders, patients and their carers are involved in their care.

2. *Risk management* – this involves risk assessment, and the way in which action is taken against identified potential risks and from actual risks through critical incidents occurring.

3. *Clinical audit* – this includes identification of areas to audit, the implementation and follow-up recommendations made.

4. *Research and education* – this includes activities which improve the patient experience and outcomes through using evidence-based practice.

5. *Staff involvement* – the approach to human resource management, staff development and performance, such as appraisals.

6. *Education, training and development* – this includes educational and training strategies and plans, along with the types of activities that are available.

7. *Information management* – this involves how information can be used to support good health care delivery, including Information Management and Technology (IMT).

ACTIVITY 8.8

Try to identify from practice, examples of the seven pillars of clinical governance in action, for example under 'patient involvement' what bodies exist which play a role in this – Patient Advice and Liaison Service (PALS).

Whilst the seven pillars are crucial in constructing a robust clinical governance framework, there have been further developments covering new national standards across health and social care. These do not replace the seven pillars, but they will be used to demonstrate progress within seven new domains of health care. They have been developed in order to meet the key principles on how health care is to be modernized, identified in the NHS Improvement Plan (DoH 2004a), and are outlined in National Standards, Local Action – Health and Social Care Standards and Planning Framework 2005/06–2007/08 (DoH 2004b). The standards are organized in seven domains, covering the full spectrum of health care defined in the Health and Social Care (Community Health and Standards) Act 2003.

The standards are described as 'core', which are non-optional, meaning all organizations must comply. In addition, there are 'developmental' standards which are broad based and provide a focus for continuous improvement over time. These standards are designed in recognition of a context in which patient expectations are increasing and will form a key part of the performance assessment arrangements by the Health care Commission. The seven domains of care in which the standards apply are

1. Safety
2. Clinical and cost effectiveness
3. Governance
4. Patient focus
5. Accessible and responsive care
6. Care environment and amenities
7. Public health

To illustrate the concept of domains of care, core and developmental standards, the following 'Patient focus' domain may be used.

Example fourth domain – patient focus

Domain outcome

Health care is provided in partnership with patients, their carers and relatives, respecting their diverse needs, preferences and choices, and in particular with other organizations (especially social care organisations) whose services impact on patient well-being.

Core standard (one of four in total in this domain)

Health care organizations have systems in place to ensure that

a) staff treat patients, their relatives and carers with dignity and respect;

b) appropriate consent is obtained when required for all contacts with patients and for the use of any patient confidential information; and

c) staff treat patient information confidentially, except where authorized by legislation to the contrary.

Related developmental standard

Health care organizations continuously improve the patient experience, based on the feedback of patients, carers and relatives.

In terms of ensuring that the arrangements are in place in local health care organizations to make effective clinical governance possible, Sale (2000) states that the following key elements are essential:

1. Quality improvement processes, such as clinical audit, are in place and integrated with the quality programme across the organization as a whole.

2. The skills of good leadership exist and are developed at the level of the clinical team.

3. Evidence-based practice is commonplace and is fully supported through the organization's systems and procedures.

4. Good practice, ideas and innovations are disseminated widely within and outside the organization.

5. High quality clinical risk reduction programmes are in place.

6. There is an open approach to the detection of adverse events which once investigated, are learnt from, and new practice is applied to avoid problems in the future.

7. Lessons obtained from complaints made by patients/relatives are learnt from and then applied in clinical practice.

8. Poor clinical performance is detected early and dealt with in order to prevent harm to other patients.

9. All professional development programmes are underpinned by clinical governance.

10. The quality of data required to monitor clinical practice is of a high standard.

11. All professional staff need to be monitored to ensure that they remain up to date with new professional and practice developments.

12. A forum for discussing all new clinical practice is established.

13. The culture of the organization and its clinical practice areas is open and participative.

14. The ethos of teamwork is well established.

15. The patient is central to care and in the relationship with health care professionals.

There are four national regulatory bodies that are currently in place to ensure that the key elements of the quality agenda are delivered. Changes will, however, take place, resulting in new and amended roles for these organizations, and so readers are advised to regularly monitor the situation in this regard. In illustrating this, the National Patient Safety Agency will be taking on board the functions of the National Clinical Assessment Authority, which will operate as a separate division with it.

The Health care Commission (CHAI) www.healthcarecommission.org.uk

Formerly known as the CHI, the full legal title of the Health care Commission is the Commission for Health care Audit and Inspection (CHAI). The role of CHAI is to promote improvement in the quality of health care in England and Wales. Within England it has the additional role of regulating the independent health care sector. CHAI has established itself as a highly influential body, carrying out clinical governance inspections and making their findings publicly available. It also has the authority to intervene when incidents and trends in poor practice are detected or reported, making recommendations on how such situations require improving. CHAI will be integrating the functions of the Mental Health Act Commission within its role. The body has a new responsibility to review complaints about the NHS which have not been resolved at a local level.

National Institute for Health and Clinical Excellence (NICE) www.nice.org.uk

NICE was established in 1999 as an independent organization, responsible for giving national guidance on the clinical and cost effectiveness of treatments and care available in the NHS. NICE is a key body in reducing the perceived inequity in the provision of treatment and services available in England and Wales. The main reason for its creation is to provide clear, evidence-based guidance about the cost-effectiveness of interventions (Baggott 2004). When such guidelines are used across the country, it should result in fewer geographical variations being encountered in the care and treatment available.

National Clinical Assessment Authority (NCAA) www.ncaa.nhs.uk

The NCAA started operating in 2001. Its job is to provide a central point of contact for the NHS when there are concerns about an individual doctor's or dentist's performance. The NCAA provides advice and carries out targeted assessments where necessary. Once an assessment has been carried out, it is then the responsibility of the employing organization, such as a health authority, primary care trust, hospital or community trust, to take the necessary action to rectify the situation.

National Patient Safety Agency (NPSA) www.npsa.nhs.uk

The NPSA was created in 2001. Its role is to oversee and collect data from the estimated 900,000 mistakes or patient safety incidents which occur each year (www.npsa.nhs.uk). In doing so, the NPSA has constructed a full single national database which records information taken from reports on incidents, such as equipment failures. Over time, this should lead to a more open culture of sharing information on adverse incidents. This can then help to ensure that mistakes are not repeated in the future. The NPSA plays a key role in making patient safety a national issue.

ACTIVITY 8.9

Take a look at the websites of the four key bodies above, and try to find examples of the work that they carry out, for example CHAI report on a hospital you are interested in.

Introduction to vignettes

The following vignettes are designed to assess your ability to identify some key issues which are relevant to clinical governance. Although each vignette is to a large extent nursing-branch specific, there are learning points to be gained from undertaking all four activities regardless of what branch is of interest to you. Read the appropriate vignette(s) and then identify the issues which are of relevance to clinical governance. You might like to use a particular reflective tool in assisting you. Additionally, discuss your findings with other students or nursing colleagues, such as your mentor in practice.

Based on adult nursing vignette

David is a 52-year-old man who has been admitted to the medical unit of a large district hospital. He was initially found in the main city park, unconscious and with a large gash on his forehead which required suturing in the emergency department, prior to his transferral to the ward. His unkempt appearance suggests that he is very probably homeless, and has been sleeping rough for some time. Shortly after admission, he regains full consciousness and is able to explain a little more about his personal circumstances, although he does appear to be rather confused and agitated. His behaviour later becomes quite abusive as he begins to use obscene language to the other patients in the four-bedded bay in which he is located. When he is challenged and reprimanded by the nurse in charge, David begins to exhibit aggressive and violent behaviour. It is suspected that this is probably due to a sense of confusion he is feeling, as the possible effects of alcohol withdrawal take hold. All the time, both other patients and staff are becoming increasingly concerned and intimidated by his presence and behaviour, and so it is decided to move him into a side room where he will be isolated. Although in the short term, this is likely to alleviate the anxieties of the other patients, the overall problems associated with David's behaviour and illness persist.

ACTIVITY 8.10

What are the clinical governance issues which as a nurse you can learn from this example?

Based on children's nursing vignette

Gary is a four-year-old boy who has recently started school. He was admitted on to the children's unit of a large district general hospital via the emergency department in order to undergo tests to determine the possible causes of a suspected febrile convulsion. During admission, Gary's mother explains that she and his father are estranged. The child will stay on the unit overnight and so his mother needs to return home briefly in order to collect some belongings required for her and Gary's stay.

After returning later that evening, the nurse on duty informs Gary's mother that he has been visited by his father. The nurse was impressed by the concern that the visitor had shown and was struck by the obvious family resemblance. The child's mother expressed alarm, explaining that it could not be his father because so far as she was aware he was working abroad. She could only conclude that the visitor in question was in fact Gary's uncle, who had been prosecuted and convicted in the past on the grounds of child abuse. Although Gary did not appear to have been adversely affected by the visit, his mother was concerned that he may have been put at risk, and lodged a formal complaint.

ACTIVITY 8.11

What are the clinical governance issues which as a nurse you can learn from this example?

Based on learning disability nursing vignette

Ellen is a 62-year-old woman who lives in an independent group home. This is the fourth home she has lived in over the past six years, apparently because of her increasingly difficult behaviour. Ellen has a moderate learning disability and requires support with her daily living skills.

Ellen has been referred to the community learning disability team because her behaviour has become increasingly aggressive, both verbally and physically. She screams for no apparent reason at staff and residents, often accusing them of hurting her and shouts that she hopes they will die. Ellen has recently started to lash out at staff and other residents. This has resulted in causing minor injuries to two female members of staff, and one elderly vulnerable resident.

Ellen has experienced a number of health problems in the past. She fell and broke her hip four years ago and often complains of discomfort. Two years ago, Ellen had a hysterectomy, after it was discovered that she had cancer. This was followed by more surgery after a further tumour was located. Ellen has found hospital visits distressing and generally presents with increased levels of anxiety and stress at such times.

Some staff are concerned that Ellen's behaviour is becoming so unmanageable that sooner or later someone is going to get seriously hurt. They are actively discussing the possibility of her having to leave and live elsewhere. It seems that every time Ellen's behaviour is perceived as being difficult she is moved on.

ACTIVITY 8.12

What are the clinical governance issues which as a nurse you can learn from this example?

Based on mental health nursing vignette

Sheila is an informal patient (i.e. not detained under the Mental Health Act) on an acute mental health admissions ward. She has made it clear that she wishes to leave the unit and has declined a request to speak to nursing or medical staff before leaving. Staff on duty feel that she should not leave the unit. As Sheila attempted to leave, staff made a decision to try to restrain her and administer intra-muscular medication against her wishes.

Sheila subsequently made a formal complaint that she had been detained against her will, falsely imprisoned and assaulted.

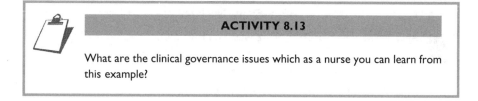

ACTIVITY 8.13

What are the clinical governance issues which as a nurse you can learn from this example?

8.8 Quality and the NMC code of professional conduct

The job of the NMC is to protect the public. This is done by ensuring that nurses, health visitors and midwives give high standards of care to their patients and clients (NMC 2004). Central to this is the 'Code of professional conduct' governing the way professionals operate (see Chapters 1 and 5).

As it is stated, the very purpose of the Code puts 'quality' at the centre of practice. Under clause 1.1 (NMC 2004), the Code is there to

- inform the professions of the standard of professional conduct required of them in the exercise of their professional accountability and practice

- inform the public, other professions and employers of the standard of professional conduct that they can expect of a registered practitioner.

In support of this, clause 1.3 (NMC 2004) requires that professionals are personally accountable for their practice. This puts the onus on individual practitioners to ensure they operate in a patient- or client-centred way. In carrying out their practice, professionals are duty bound by the Code to cooperate with other members of the multi-disciplinary team, to maintain their knowledge base and level of competence, and to identify and minimize risk to patients and clients.

8.9 Conclusion

Quality as a concept is a dominant feature of organizational life across the world of health and social care. True to the principles of TQM, this is being driven from the top in terms of policy initiatives announced by the Department of Health, which are then implemented at the local level. TQM also insists that everyone involved in patient or client care has a role to play, thereby taking personal ownership of what and how they do things. In guiding how you operate as a quality-orientated practitioner, your employing organization's clinical governance framework will assist and direct you. This will include action to ensure risks are avoided, adverse events are rapidly detected, openly investigated and lessons learned. Furthermore, good practice should be rapidly disseminated and systems put in place to ensure continuous improvements in clinical care (Cook 1998). The content and activities covered in this chapter will provide you with some valuable insights as to how this can be achieved. This will ensure that you operate as a fully engaged professional with quality being central to your practice.

═══ SELF-EVALUATION ═══

? And, finally, your chance to revise what you have learnt from this chapter

1. How would you define quality care?

2. Which groups have an interest in quality care?

3. What are Maxwell's (1992) six dimensions of quality?

4. What do you understand by 'patient-centred care'?

5. How would you define TQM?

6. What is meant by a 'zero-defects' approach?

7. What are the seven pillars of clinical governance?

8. What is the main purpose of each – CHAI, NICE, NCAA, NPSA?

9. Why is quality important to you as a professional practitioner?

References

Baggott, R. (2004) *Health and Health Care in Britain* (Third edition). Palgrave Macmillan, Basingstoke.

Bloor, K. and Maynard, A. (1998) *Clinical Governance: Clinician, Heal Thyself?* IHSM, London.

Carruthers, I. and Holland, P. (1991) Quality assurance – choice for the individual. *International Journal of Health Care Quality Assurance* 4(2): 9–17.

Commission for Health Improvement (CHI) (2003) www.healthcarecommission.org.uk

Cook, R. (1998) Picture in profile – clinical governance. *Health Service Journal* 9 July: 26–27.

Crosby, P.B. (1984) *Quality Without Tears*. McGraw-Hill, New York.

Deming, W.E. (1986) *Out of the Crisis*. Cambridge University Press, Cambridge.

Department of Health (DoH) (1991) *The Patient's Charter*. HMSO, London.

Department of Health (DoH) (1997) *The New NHS: Modern, Dependable*. The Stationery Office, London.

Department of Health (DoH) (1998) *A First Class Service*. The Stationery Office, London.

Department of Health (DoH) (2000) *The NHS Plan: A Plan for Investment, a Plan for Reform*. The Stationery Office, London.

Department of Health (DoH) (2001) *Learning from Bristol: The Report of the Public Inquiry into Children's Heart Surgery at the Bristol Royal Infirmary 1984–95*. The Stationery Office, London.

Department of Health (DoH) (2004a) *The NHS Improvement Plan*. The Stationery Office, London.

Department of Health (DoH) (2004b) *National Standards, Local Action – Health and Social Care Standards and Planning Framework 2005/6–2007/8*. The Stationery Office, London.

Department of Health and Social Security (DHSS) (1983) *NHS Management Inquiry (The Griffiths Management Report)*. DHSS, London.

Henderson, E. (1998) *Managing for Quality*. Open University, Milton Keynes.

Hewison, A. (2004) *Management for Nurses and Health Professionals*. Blackwell, Oxford.

Juran, J.M. (1986) The quality trilogy. *Quality Progress* 19(8): 19–24.

Kendall, L. and Lissauer, R. (2003) *The Future Health Worker*. IPPR, London.

Kennedy, I. (2001) *The Inquiry into the Management of Care of Children Receiving Complex Heart Surgery at the Bristol Royal Infirmary 1984–1995*. Central Office of Information, Bristol.

Klein, R. (2001) *The New Politics of the NHS* (Fourth edition). Prentice Hall, London.

Maxwell, R.J. (1992) Dimensions of quality revisited: From thought to action. *Quality in Health Care* 1: 171–177.

McSherry, R. and Pearce, P. (2002) *Clinical Governance: A Guide to Implementation for Health Care Professionals*. Blackwell Science, Oxford.

Morris, B. (1989) Total quality management. *International Journal of Health Care Quality Assurance* 2(3): 4–6.

National Patient Safety Agency (NPSA) www.npsa.nhs.uk

Nursing and Midwifery Council (NMC) (2004) *Code of Professional Conduct*. NMC, London.

Oakland, J. (1993) *Total Quality Management* (Second edition). Butterworth-Heinemann, Oxford.

Øvretveit, J. (1992) *Health Service Quality*. Blackwell Science, Oxford.

Parsley, K. and Corrigan, P. (1999) *Quality Improvement in Health Care: Putting Evidence into Practice* (Second edition). Stanley Thornes, Cheltenham.

Royal Berkshire and Battle Hospitals NHS Trust (2004) www.rbbn.nhs.uk

Sale, D. (2000) *Quality Assurance: A Pathway to Excellence*. Macmillan, Basingstoke.

Scally, G. and Donaldson, L. (1998) Clinical governance and the drive for quality improvement in the new NHS in England. *British Medical Journal* 317: 61–65.

Wanless, D. (2002) Securing our future health: Taking a long term view – final report. HM Treasury, London.

Williamson, J.W. (1978) Formulating priorities for quality assurance activity: Description of its method and its application. *Journal of the American Medical Association* 239: 631–637.

Suggested reading

Marquis, B.L. and Huston, C.J. (2003) *Leadership Roles and Management Functions in Nursing: Theory and Application* (Fourth edition). Lippincott, Philadelphia.

This is a good general text for students of health care management, which contains some activities to help consolidate learning.

Parsley, K. and Corrigan, P. (1994) *Quality Improvement in Nursing and Health care: A Practical Approach*. Chapman and Hall, London.

Sale, D. (1996) *Quality Assurance; for Nurses and Other Members of the Health Care Team* (Second edition). Macmillan, Basingstoke.

These two texts are seminal pieces of literature on the subject of quality in a health care context, providing a valuable theoretical resource.

Swage, T. (2001) *Clinical Governance in Health Care Practice.* Butterworth-Heinemann, Oxford.

Wright, J. and Hill, P. (2003) *Clinical Governance.* Churchill Livingstone, London.

These two texts will provide a fuller theoretical basis for what clinical governance is about as an all-embracing quality assurance system for health care services.

CHAPTER 9

Leadership for Practice

Yvette Cox and Andrée le May

CONTENTS

- Defining leadership
- Leadership qualities
- Leadership theories
- Motivation theories
- Evaluation

LEARNING OUTCOMES

This chapter should enable you to

- Discuss the complexities of leading teams of people working in health care
- Detail some of the qualities that are required to lead contemporary health
- Consider how you function as a leader yourself
- Analyse how you might evaluate your own and other's styles of leadership

9.1 Introduction

Leadership is a multifaceted and complex aspect of professional life that has become increasingly important within the nursing professions over the last

20 years. This prominence is partly a response to a perceived need to create leaders from within the disciplines of nursing and midwifery, and partly as a result of working in health/social care services where uncertainty, complexity and continuous change are the hallmarks of day-to-day practice. These, when taken together, call for the creation of a nursing and midwifery workforce that is able to adapt to rapid change, inspirationally develop practice and evaluate the impact of altered practices on the quality of care that is provided – in other words a workforce where leadership and team-working are dominant.

Additionally, recent major leadership failures have been identified as significant factors in the breakdown of health and social care in general. In their response to the Bristol Inquiry (Kennedy 2001), the Department of Health (2001) recommended guidance from the NHS Leadership Centre on acceptable leadership practice and style suggesting that an emphasis be placed on, for example:

- Leadership from the top

- Empowerment of staff

- Team work

- Prevention, rather than correction of adverse outcomes; analysing, simplifying and improving processes

- Commitment to encouraging clinicians into management; ensuring greater involvement of women and people from ethnic minority backgrounds in management

- And a strong patient focus.

(DoH 2001: 83–84)

This, reinforced by the earlier reforms stipulated in the NHS Plan (DoH 2000), led to an increase in interest in leadership and the training that leaders required in order to deliver high quality services within a changing health care system.

Whilst we can track the positioning of leadership both within the NHS and the nursing professions as gaining prominence over the last 15 years, the concept of leadership remains hard to define and therefore develop in people. Leadership means different things to different people and although there have been numerous research studies which have looked at the different types of leadership, none has come up with a definition that captures leadership in its totality. Despite this uncertainty we hope that this chapter will provide you with a greater understanding of the complexities of leadership.

9.2 Defining leadership

Leadership, although it is something that we talk about and recognise as desirable within both people and organisations, is hard to define. This is probably because it is difficult to separate the concept of leadership from the jobs that leaders do and the ways in which they do them. Most definitions of leadership originate from researcher's observations of how leaders behave and how people react to these behaviours. Before reading on, write a sentence yourself which sets out what you think leadership means then compare your definition with the ones that we have given you in Box 9.1.

BOX 9.1 Defining leadership

Kouzes and Posner (1997: 36) state: 'The word "lead" at its root means "go travel, guide"'.

Northouse (2004: 3) defines leadership as '. . . a process whereby an individual influences a group of individuals to achieve a common goal'.

As you can see from these definitions leadership is an interactive process which is about leading people (most frequently referred to as followers) in order to undertake a project/task or develop an idea. The relationship between leaders and followers is fundamental – since a leader directs others to achieve specific goals (tasks/targets) and in doing so influences the followers (and is influenced by the followers) in a variety of different ways. The interrelationship between leaders and followers is fundamental since a leader without followers cannot lead and a group without a leader lacks direction. The group (i.e. the leader and the followers) therefore provides the context within which leadership takes place.

9.3 Leadership qualities

The literature frequently refers to leadership qualities (Daft 1999, Alimo-Metcalfe and Alban-Metcalfe 2002, NHS Leadership Centre 2002) that help leaders to be effective both in influencing and guiding others. These qualities include:

- Having vision and being able to communicate it to others
- Motivating others
- Being honest, credible and trustworthy
- Responsiveness and flexibility
- Being innovative
- Being able to think creatively
- Having charisma
- Having good communication skills
- Being able to work across boundaries (e.g. between health and social care)
- Having a variety of personal resources and energy to be a leader.

Table 9.1 Types of power

Position power	A ward sister/charge nurse has authority and responsibility for the ward and as such their power is because of their position within the hierarchy of the organisation and their profession. This gives them the right to expect others to comply with their wishes and to influence the hiring and firing of staff.
Personal power	This is also known as charismatic power and is associated with being able to inspire and enthuse people. Personal power is not always associated with position.
Expert power	If a member of the team is acknowledged as an expert in their field others will come to them for help and advice. This form of power works most effectively when the expert freely shares their knowledge and skills with others.
Resource power	Power is linked to the ability to reward people through the use of resources – e.g. rewarding members of the team by praising them; letting them go home early; awarding off-duty requests and providing funding for individuals to attend courses and study days.

Source: Adapted from French and Raven (1959).

But in addition to these, leaders may need to use their power to influence people and policy or decision-making committees. What do we mean by power? There are four main sources of power that a leader may use to influence individuals or their team (Table 9.1).

The leader's power will only be effective if the team members acknowledge it (Boddy and Paton 1998) and respect the leader. However, sometimes leaders exert their power unequally favouring some team members over others; in these instances the leader will not gain the team's respect and as a consequence will find it difficult to convince team members of the value of their contribution or the work of the group. This may manifest itself as grudging compliance that in turn results in poor performance. A leader has to learn to use their power appropriately in order to achieve the desired outcomes.

As we review the different theories of leadership in the following section, the power base of the leader will be identified.

9.4 Leadership theories

Each of the theories outlined within this chapter has been written from a different perspective and together they provide a greater understanding of leadership and provide insight into the complexity of successful leadership.

Trait theory

One of the first attempts to study leadership was at the beginning of the twentieth century when researchers began to be interested in identifying the traits that made some people great leaders. Fascination with this approach to understanding leadership continued throughout that century (e.g. Stodgill 1948, Mann 1959 and more recently Bass 1990) with the focus of these studies being placed entirely on the leader – followers or the situations in which the leaders worked were not taken into account. The resultant belief was that leaders were born and not made, and that leaders had some superior characteristics that differentiated them from other people. These traits included:

- Greater intelligence
- More self-confidence
- Determination
- Integrity
- Sociability.

The trait theories became known as the 'great man' theories because they focused on identifying characteristics that great male political and military leaders possessed. Women, at the time, did not occupy many leadership roles and were therefore omitted from this debate. The power base of this type of leader was seen as their personal qualities.

Whilst this type of approach to understanding leadership – on its own – is now seen as naïve, several writers on leadership continue to highlight leadership characteristics that are most admired by followers therefore adding credibility to the idea that leadership traits are important aspects of successful leading (see for instance the leadership qualities identified above). For example, Kouzes and Posner (1995) identified four frequently recorded traits which we would all value in leaders – being honest, competent, forward looking and inspirational.

Despite shortcomings, the trait theory does enable leaders to assess their strengths and to identify areas in which they need to develop further to enhance their leadership. It is important to recognise that a leader may not inherently possess all of the qualities identified, and that some leadership skills can be learnt.

One major factor that was not taken into consideration within the trait theories was the impact that the behaviour of a leader has on the followers. Lewin and Lippitt (1938) identified that individuals tended to have different approaches or styles of leadership that they developed to meet the needs of their followers and the work that they were doing.

Styles theory

The styles approach examined what leaders did and how they acted towards their followers. Stodgill (1974) found that a leader's behaviour depended on whether the leader focused on either organising work, defining roles and responsibilities, scheduling work activities (Stodgill called this *initiating structure*); or on building camaraderie, respect, trust and liking between the leader and followers (Stodgill called this *consideration*).

Table 9.2 outlines the broad classification of the styles of leadership that emerged (Mullins 1999).

Table 9.2 Classification of styles of leadership

	Authoritarian Style	**Democratic Style**	**Laissez-faire Style**
Primary focus	The work to be done. Completing the task to a high standard. Maintaining power and control over the work.	Development of individuals and the team. Delegation used as a means to develop others.	Enabling others to manage and control their own work.
Focus of power	The leader	The team	Individual members of the team
Normal behaviour	Initiating structure by defining roles and responsibilities for all team members. Planning the work to be undertaken each day. Making decisions and expecting others to follow directions given.	Sharing leadership functions amongst the team. Acting as part of the team. Seeking opinions of staff in the decision-making process. Interacting with all members of the group.	Allowing individuals to work autonomously and only assisting individuals when required.
Leaders' expectations of others	Feedback from staff on progress of work. Refer/check decisions with the leader.	Take on responsibility and develop skills.	Work autonomously. Request assistance when required.

ACTIVITY 9.1

Consider the impact that these different styles of leaders might have on the staff working with them. Draw on examples from your own practice to help you.

9.5 The impact of the leader's style upon staff

Authoritarian style

Junior members of staff often feel secure with this style of leadership because they are being directed and know that they can turn to someone who will make decisions and guide them. However, if the leader is absent some work may not be undertaken because members of staff are not used to organising their own work and may be unsure about the decisions to be made.

As staff develop their knowledge and skills and become more experienced they may find this style increasingly frustrating as they are not learning how to plan and direct work activities and make decisions themselves. The lack of emphasis on developing staff within the team may also result in the team not working well together – especially when the leader is not present to direct activities.

Democratic style

The democratic leader delegates aspects of their role to members of the team (i.e.) gives 'another the authority to undertake specific actions or decisions' (Boddy and Paton 1998: 157), and in so doing develops the knowledge and skills of team members. Box 9.2 gives examples of how leaders make delegation effective.

BOX 9.2 Effective delegation

1. *Recognising the abilities of the person to whom the work is being delegated –* choosing the right person to delegate the work to is essential if the leader retains responsibility for their actions

2. *Agreeing what is to be done and to what standard –* giving the individual the necessary authority and responsibility to undertake the task

3. *Willingness to trust that individual to do the job –* the leader should monitor performance without undue interference

4. *Commitment to develop skills in members of the team –* if the person has never undertaken the task before they will need to be shown what is expected of them

5. *Gaining satisfaction from knowing that others can do the job as well –* acknowledging that others may be able to do the job better than you can.

Members of staff working with the democratic leader develop skills in decision-making and leading the team. The emphasis on team working means that the camaraderie develops and the team can function in the absence of the leader. Junior members of the team may require more direction initially. Some members of the team however may prefer the leader to make decisions and may feel uncomfortable with this approach perhaps preferring a more autocratic approach.

Laissez-faire style

This style is better suited to working with followers who are experienced and capable of taking on responsibility rather than those who are more junior and still require direction and support.

Most individuals do have a preferred leadership style that they like to work with. Where employee-centred styles of leadership (democratic and laissez-faire) have been observed staff have been found to be more content, turnover rates lower and job satisfaction higher than when more autocratic approaches have been used. Leaders also have preferred styles – many preferring the democratic approach. The democratic style of leadership, however, is not appropriate to every circumstance and leaders need to be able to alter their leadership style to suit the circumstances they are faced with as you will see when you read the next section.

Contingency theory

The basis of contingency theory is that effective leaders were able to select the most appropriate leadership style according to the needs and characteristics of their followers and the demands of the situation (Fielder 1967).

ACTIVITY 9.2

What factors do you think a leader should take into account in order to ensure they are using the most appropriate leadership style?

Some of the factors given below will be the same as the ones that you have listed. They fall broadly into two categories – the needs and characteristics of staff and the demands of the situation.

1. **Needs and characteristics of staff**

   Within a team of health and social care professionals there will be people at varying stages of their career and personal development. In order to get the best out of each person (and the team as a whole), the leader needs to take into account certain factors when considering the most appropriate leadership style to use (see Table 9.3).

2. **Demands of the situation**

   Three main factors influence the style of leadership adopted when undertaking any work activity (see Table 9.3). These are:

   a. *The nature of the task*: Emergency situations require a different approach from normal day-to-day activities. With complex tasks or work that has never been undertaken before, the leader needs to obtain different views as to the best way of achieving the task.

   b. *The timescale in which to complete the task*: The more urgent a task is the less time a leader has to involve others in decision-making and planning the task.

Table 9.3 Factors which may influence the adoption of a leadership style

Factors	Characteristics	Preferred Leadership Style
The ability of the staff	New and inexperienced staff Experienced staff	Authoritarian Democratic/Laissez faire
Willingness of staff	Unwilling Willing	Authoritarian Democratic/Laissez faire
The nature of the task	Emergency Complex task	Authoritarian Democratic
The timescale within which to complete the task	Short timescale Long timescale	Authoritarian Democratic/Laissez faire
The consequences of not being successful	High risk/low risk	Depends on the leader and the staff involved in the task

c. *The consequences of not being successful*: This is a complex aspect to consider. If there is a risk to patients or the quality of service provided if the task is not carried out successfully the leader is more likely to want to be prescriptive in what has to be done and how it will be carried out. On the other hand, the leader may want to gain opinion and assistance from others to minimise the risks involved.

The contingency theory highlights that it is not appropriate to use one style of leadership all of the time and that leaders need to be able to adopt the most appropriate style for both the situation and the individual staff members that they are leading.

Although Fielder's (1967) research on contingency theory emphasised that the leader needed to consider the willingness of staff when deciding on an appropriate style, it did not examine the impact that leaders might have on motivating staff. Recent writings on leadership (e.g. NHS Leadership Centre 2002 and Daft 1999) pay particular attention to the importance of motivation if leaders are to be successful in completing the task and also developing their followers.

9.6 Motivation

What is motivation?

Motivation causes a person to act in a particular way and can be classified as either extrinsic (e.g. pay, fringe benefits, pension, security) or intrinsic (e.g. feelings of pride and achievement, liking the work itself, personal growth, learning on the job). Many different features of motivation have been described and are summarised in Table 9.4.

There are numerous theories of motivation, all of which go some way to explaining what it is, but there is no one theory that fully explains this phenomenon. One common mistake that leaders make is to assume that all staff work towards the same goal and that they are all willing to co-operate with one another to achieve that goal. Think back to your own experiences of working with people and it will be clear that different things motivate different people in different ways. To help you to understand how complex motivation is and how leaders might use knowledge of motivation theory to help them motivate teams, we have highlighted a few of the major theories below.

Table 9.4 Features of motivation

Motivation is unique to the individual	What motivates one person may not motivate another
Motivation is usually intentional	The individual has a choice of whether to act or not
Motivation is multifaceted	No single thing has been identified as being able to motivate every individual. The two most important aspects to consider are: 1. What gets a person in a 'ready state' to do something 2. What makes an individual engage in an activity

Maslow's hierarchy of needs

Maslow's theory (1970) was based on the premise that people always want more, and that what they want is dependent on what they already have. He suggested that human needs are arranged in a hierarchy and that once a lower need has been satisfied it no longer acts as a strong motivator and the individual can then seek to satisfy the needs in the next level of the hierarchy (see Table 9.5).

Maslow did emphasise that the hierarchy was not a fixed order, and that for some people there may be a reversal in the hierarchy so that they may strive for self-actualisation at the expense of some of the lower-order needs. It is also clear that some people are satisfied with the lower-order needs being met and do not strive for more.

When we apply Maslow's theory to work we need to take a number of factors into account:

1. People do not necessarily meet all of their needs through work. Some people work to gain a salary to support their hobby, which in turn satisfies their higher-order needs.

2. People place different values on needs, and the amount of value placed on a need may change over time.

3. People at the same level within the hierarchy do not necessarily have the same motivational factors – there are different ways to achieve what you want.

4. Job satisfaction does not always lead to improved performance at work.

This might help us to understand more as he suggests that rather than being motivated to do something because of its positive effects, we might feel motivated to stop doing something because of its negative effects.

Table 9.5 Maslow's hierarchy of needs and its potential application to work life

Levels in Maslow's Hierarchy (1 being most basic – 5 being most sophisticated)	Components of Each Level of the Hierarchy	Aspects of Work Life that Could Fit with Each Level in Maslow's Hierarchy
1. Physiological needs	Food, water, sex, sleep	Pay, good working conditions
2. Safety needs	Security, stability, protection	Safe working conditions, job security, benefits
3. Social needs	Love, affection, belonging	Cohesive group, friendly, good team working
4. Esteem needs	Self-respect, prestige, status	Job title, high status role
5. Self-actualisation needs	Growth, advancement, creativity	Challenging job, achievement, opportunity for creativity

Herzberg's (1987) two factor theory of motivation

Herzberg (1987) developed his theory of motivation by asking people to identify times when they felt exceptionally good or bad about their current job. The results clustered into two sets of factors that might affect motivation at work (hygiene factors and motivational or growth factors) (see Figure 9.1).

1. Hygiene factors related to the job context and environment and caused dissatisfaction with work. He concluded that if leaders paid proper attention to these factors (e.g. pay, working conditions), they would be able to prevent dissatisfaction amongst the team, but that these would not motivate the individual.

2. Motivational or growth factors all related to the job and the content of work itself. Herzberg concluded that these were stronger motivating factors than the hygiene factors and that in order to motivate an individual the leader should give proper attention to these aspects.

Both Maslow's and Herzberg's work centred on what motivates an individual. Other theories of motivation (e.g. Vroom's) have looked at the process of motivation for example how behaviour is initiated, directed and sustained. Exploring the combination of all of these approaches is probably the best way to explain the complexity of leading and following people.

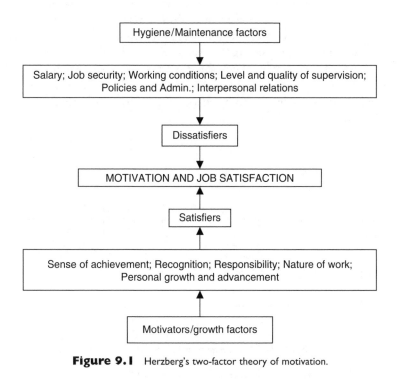

Figure 9.1 Herzberg's two-factor theory of motivation.

Vroom's (1964) expectancy theory of motivation

Expectancy theory is based on the premise that an individual will be motivated if they feel that the effort they will have to put into a job will be rewarded by something that they value. An individual is unlikely to put in the effort required if they think that the objectives of the job are unclear, they have not the ability to do the task, or if they do not have the materials they need to do the job well (see Figure 9.2).

Vroom's expectancy theory of motivation fits well with the transactional theory of leadership (Burns 1978). Transactional leaders often influence the behaviour of their staff by bargaining with them; they agree to provide rewards in exchange for staff undertaking specific work (Burns 1978). The power of the transactional manager is based on their ability to award rewards (resource power), the transactional leader clarifies organisational rewards and punishments, and monitors the performance of the staff. If the member of staff behaves in a way that is desired by the leader, and achieves the specified outcome, they receive rewards that they value (Bass 1985).

Transformational leadership on the other hand embodies many of the positive aspects of all of the motivational theories described above. Transformational leadership is described as 'a process that changes and transforms individuals' (Northouse 2004: 169) (see Table 9.6 for an outline of the characteristics of transformational leaders).

Transformational leaders encourage followers to strive towards a common goal leaving their self-interests aside; they constantly review and improve services and care as well as inspiring their team to do likewise. They do this by using a combination of power sources (see Table 9.1) to influence the team in various ways. For example using personal power may get the team to identify with them and want to work with them whereas their expertise may inspire others to improve practice and to make a difference. Additionally, the transformational leader motivates their team by enabling them to gain intrinsic satisfaction (reward) from their work.

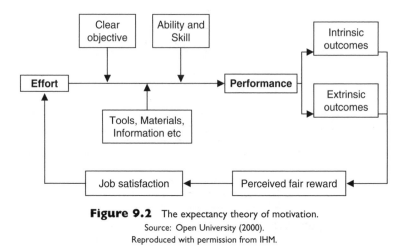

Figure 9.2 The expectancy theory of motivation.
Source: Open University (2000).
Reproduced with permission from IHM.

Table 9.6 Characteristics of the transformational leader

Inspirational	They can describe what the majority of people want for the future in such a way that the specific actions and objectives to be achieved are clear, so people feel that the vision is achievable.
Charismatic	Transformational leaders arouse strong positive emotions in followers who identify with the leader and want to emulate them. They can influence the values, beliefs and behaviour of followers (Zalesnik 1989).
Intellectual stimulation	The leader increases followers' awareness of problems and stimulates them to view problems from new perspectives and to seek solutions.
Individualised consideration	Support and encouragement is provided to individual staff that are provided with learning opportunities and enabled to develop.

Source: Bass and Avolio (1994).

It is little wonder then that transformational leadership is currently popular within the NHS as this approach fits well with the Labour government's objectives to modernise and reform health care whilst putting patients at the centre of care (DoH 2000). If we are to achieve this level of transformation then we need adaptable leaders who are able to identify different and better ways of working, solve problems quickly, be responsible for decision-taking and inspire others to transform practice (McNichol 2002).

Problem solving and decision-taking

Problem solving is a process that culminates in a decision being made and is an essential leadership skill. During the process of problem solving and decision-taking, it is important that the individual keeps an open mind and does not jump to a conclusion too early on without thoroughly exploring the problem and the factors that are contributing to it occurring (see Table 9.7).

This may seem a lengthy and complicated process to solving problems and make sound decisions, but as Einstein once said 'You can't solve a problem with the same thinking that created it' (Bercovitz 2001).

9.7 Evaluating leadership

Considerable attention is being focused on measuring performance within health and social care – either as a contribution to the running of an effective service or as a way to help individuals see how well they are doing something (e.g. through appraisal or individual performance review). Measuring the effectiveness of leaders (i.e. their ability to lead changes and teams of people) is just as important to the smooth running of organisations providing care as measuring other more tangible aspects of care, for example the numbers of people waiting beyond a specified length of time in Accident and Emergency Departments or for surgery.

There are many different ways to evaluate leadership performance but they can be broadly grouped into approaches which are self-reflective (i.e. you think

Table 9.7 Stages of problem solving and decision-taking

Analyse the problem	This aspect of problem solving is often overlooked. The problem solver often jumps through the stages of problem solving and decides on the solution to the problem without fully investigating the factors contributing to the problem. By doing this they may arrive at the wrong decision and not solve the problem but compound it further. To avoid this it is useful to consider: 1. Why is there a problem? 2. How does the problem manifest itself? 3. What additional information needs to be known?
State the objectives you want to achieve in solving the problem	This stage is important because it clarifies what you are trying to achieve in solving the problem. Ask yourself 1. What do you want to achieve? 2. What timescale do you want to achieve this in? 3. What other factors must you consider?
Generate as many solutions to the problem as possible	By identifying many different solutions to the problem, the problem solver will be able to combine/or select from those that most closely meet the need.
Evaluate the solutions against the objectives	Evaluate each of the potential solutions to the problem to see which most closely meets the objectives that you identified.
Decision-taking	The final stage of problem solving is decision-taking. At this point the individual decides on the course of action to be taken.

Source: Open University (2000).

about your ability to lead and the ways in which you do this and identify your strengths and limitations) or ways that draw on other people's perceptions of your ability to lead (e.g. a line manager's or team members' perceptions).

Self-reflective techniques for measuring leadership performance

One approach to the evaluation of leadership performance is to measure your own performance. This will involve you reflecting on your achievements, your style and how other people react to you (see Chapter 3). You might use a list of questions to help you to structure your evaluations or simply think about how you are performing. Daft (1999) provides, at the end of most chapters in his book, questions that you can ask yourself about the ways in which you lead change and teams. For instance, at the end of his chapter (pp. 260–261) on motivation he suggests some questions about how important you feel certain things are to motivating your team. This includes assigning a numerical value of importance (1 is not important through to 7 being very important):

The feeling of self-esteem a person gets from being in the job.
The opportunity for personal growth and development in the job
The feeling of security in the job
The feeling of worthwhile accomplishment in the job.

He then provides a formula for you to use to make an assessment of abilities to meet your team members' needs of security, esteem, autonomy and self-actualization.

There are many similar questionnaires and self-assessment tools that you might like to try out to see just how successful a leader you are. However, one of the problems with these sorts of approaches is that you might think you score well as a leader but the people that you lead may disagree. So in addition to your own reflections you might like to try asking others what they think!

Techniques for gaining feedback from other people about your ability to lead

The feedback process in general is one in which another person (or people) watch you lead (perhaps your manager or another colleague) or experience your leadership through being a team member and then report back to you how they feel about it. This process allows them to observe your style of leadership over a period of time, make an assessment of it (either just through their observation or by filling out questionnaires), and talk to you about it, therefore allowing you to decide how you might develop your skills further. One popular example of this is known as 360-degree feedback.

360-degree feedback is a technique that involves systematically asking other people, in confidence, about their perceptions of your performance. It is a relatively simple thing to do and will provide you with useful pointers for improvement as well as reassurances about the good aspects of your performance. There is no single way of doing this – you can either ask people to tell you or write about your performance or get them to fill out a questionnaire or other types of framework. A good example for you to look up would be the 360-degree assessment framework that accompanies the leadership qualities framework (NHS Leadership Centre 2004 – at their website www.nhsleadershipqualities.nhs.uk/assessment.asp).

There are several advantages to this approach as well as disadvantages. The advantages for the person being assessed include:

- becoming more aware of your leadership style

- being able to reflect on your strengths and weaknesses

- having someone else tell you about how you lead and maybe show you, through the assessment, things that you are unaware of

- as a result of the feedback having the opportunity to design a self-development plan that allows you to take control and responsibility for enhancing your leadership abilities.

There are other advantages related to organisational development which result from this – such as

- improved communication between people at different levels in the organisation

- the creation of an environment in which people are more willing to share their perceptions of others positively

■ increased understanding of how leaders function in teams and how team members (followers) can contribute to this.

Despite these advantages, there are some disadvantages for both the person being assessed and the organisation, which include:

■ poorly communicated feedback which is more destructive than positive

■ the identification of development needs which then cannot be supported by the organisation (or the team).

9.8 Conclusion

Leadership is about having realistic vision, inspiring others to subscribe to that vision and then enabling them to create it. This chapter was designed to help you to learn more about this complex aspect of professional life and as a result of that to be better equipped to lead teams more confidently in the future, change practice as a result of that, evaluate the success or failure of these interventions and celebrate the successes that you and your team share through those experiences.

SELF-EVALUATION

And, finally, your chance to revise what you have learnt from this chapter

■ Which styles of leadership have you experienced in terms of being a follower and in terms of being a leader?

■ In relation to delegation, what responsibilities have been delegated to you? How did the 'leader' monitor your performance?

■ What motivates you as a student nurse to practise safely and effectively?

■ Review the four characteristics of the transformational leader and discuss with a friend or colleague why you think this type of leadership is popular in the NHS?

■ Read Daft's (1999) chapter on the self-reflective questions for measuring leadership performance and apply them to yourself.

References

Alimo-Metcalfe, B. and Alban-Metcalfe, J. (2002) Half the battle. *Health Service Journal* 112(5795): 26–27.

Bass, B. (1985). *Leadership and Performance beyond Expectations*. Free Press, New York.

Bass, B. (1990) *Bass and Stogdill's Handbook of Leadership: A Survey of Theory and Research*. Free Press, New York.

Bass, M. and Avolio, B. (1994) *Improving Organisational Effectiveness through Transformational Leadership*. Sage, Thousand Oaks.

Bercovitz, A. (2001) *Problem Solve like Einstein*. Vista CA [Online] 25th August 2004. http://www.einsteinalive.com/page.php?page=probsolv.

Boddy, D. and Paton, R. (1998) *Management. An Introduction.* Prentice Hall, Harlow.

Burns, J. (1978) *Leadership.* Harper and Row, New York.

Daft, R. (1999) *Leadership: Theory and Practice.* The Dryden Press, Fort Worth.

Department of Health (DoH) (2000) *The NHS Plan.* HMSO, London.

Department of Health (DoH) (2001) The Department of Health's Response to the Report of the Public Inquiry into children's heart surgery at the Bristol Royal Infirmary 1984–1995. Department of Health, London.

Fielder, F. (1967) *A Theory of Leadership Effectiveness.* McGraw Hill, New York.

French, J. and Raven, B. (1959) The basis of social power. In: Cartwright, D. (ed.) *Studies in Social Power.* Institute for Social Research, Ann Arbour.

Herzberg, F. (1987). One more time: How do you motivate employees? *Harvard Business Review* 1: 65, September/October.

Kennedy, I. (2001) *The Report of the Inquiry into Children's Heart Surgery at the Bristol Royal Infirmary 1984–1995: Learning from Bristol,* HMSO, London.

Kouzes, J. and Posner, B. (1995) *The Leadership Challenge.* Jossey-Bass, San Francisco.

Lewin, K. and Lippitt, R. (1938) An experimental approach to the study of autocracy and democracy: A preliminary note. *Sociometry* 1: 292–300.

Mann, R. (1959) A review of the relationship between personality and performance in small groups. *Psychology Bulletin* 56: 241–270.

Maslow, A. (1970) *Motivation and Personality* (Second edition). Harper and Row, New York.

McNichol, E. (2002) Thinking outside the box. *Nursing Management* 9: 4 July.

Mullins, L. (1999) *Management and Organisational Behaviour* (Fifth edition). Prentice Hall, Harlow.

NHS Leadership Centre (2002) *The NHS Leadership Qualities Framework.* Department of Health, London.

NHS Leadership Centre (2004) The 360 degree Assessment. www.nhsleadershipqualities.nhs.uk/assessment.asp.

Northouse, P. (2004) *Leadership: Theory and Practice.* Sage, London.

Open University (2000) *Managing in Health and Social Care.* The Open University, Milton Keynes.

Stodgill, R. (1948) Personal factors associated with leadership: A survey of the literature. *Journal of Psychology* 25: 31–71.

Stodgill, R. (1974) *Manual for the Leader Behaviour Description Questionnaire form XII.* Bureau of Business Research, Ohio State University.

Vroom, V. (1964) *Work and Motivation.* Wiley, New York.

Zalesnik, A. (1992) Managers and leaders: Are they different? *Harvard Business Review* 70: 126–135.

📖 Suggested reading

Daft, R. (1999) *Leadership: Theory and Practice.* The Dryden Press, Fort Worth.
This is a sound basic text which is easy to read and is applied to health and social care practices. Apart from the useful self-assessment questions, this text also focuses on the role of followers and therefore provides valuable information for leaders and followers.

Northouse, P. (2004). *Leadership: Theory and Practice.* Sage, London.
This popular, easy to read book offers description and application of several approaches to leadership. Its strength is its emphasis on practical advice and how to apply approaches/techniques to practice.

Evidence-Based Practice and Clinical Effectiveness

CHAPTER 10

Evidence-Based Practice

Lorraine Ireland

CONTENTS

- Definitions of Evidence-Based Practice (EBP)

- Clinical Effectiveness

- Benefits of EBP, the concept of 'best evidence'

- Research and its relationship to EBP

- Research paradigms

- Hierarchies of evidence

- Asking questions and finding evidence

- Individual client needs and professional judgement

LEARNING OUTCOMES

This chapter should enable you to

- Define the term 'Evidence-Based Practice' and its relationship to Clinical Effectiveness

- Review the benefits of evidence-based practice

- Explore the relationship between evidence-based practice and clinical effectiveness

- Examine the concept of research and its interface with evidence-based practice

■ Explore how the choice of research paradigm influences the evidence gained

■ Understand the influence of hierarchies of evidence on the concept of 'best evidence'

■ Understand how the pursuit of evidence-based practice relates to asking practice-related questions

■ Recognize the centrality of individual client needs and professional judgement to the pursuit of evidence-based practice

10.1 Introduction

'Evidence-based care' has become a widely used term and practitioners in all health care professions are urged to base their care on evidence. Part of being a professional is having claim to a distinct body of knowledge which informs practice and which together with a regulated period of education justifies public confidence (see Chapter 1). This chapter examines the evidence-based health care movement considering its origin and definition. Models for evidence-based practice are then considered. The interface between evidence-based practice and research is then explored in order to consider the contribution that research can make to evidence-based care. It will be shown that research is one of many forms of evidence for practice. To understand how research can develop evidence, some understanding is required of how philosophy informs methodological choices. It will be seen that the pursuit of what constitutes 'best evidence' is fraught with tensions relating to values and beliefs. These challenges are explored in order to help you understand how evidence-based health care is a critical process in which professional judgement is integrated with consideration of the needs and wishes of our clients. It will be shown that to incorporate all of these aspects, practitioners must ask client-centred questions that arise from practice. In this way the evidence-based process can be used to develop and justify our caring practices.

10.2 What is evidence-based practice?

Informing many definitions of evidence-based practice in nursing are themes found within definitions of evidence-based medicine. The evidence-based medicine movement in the United Kingdom had its origins in the early 1980s when concern was raised about the variety and diversity of treatments offered to clients despite them sharing the same fundamental problems. The best-known definition is that of Sackett *et al.* (1996: 71) which highlights key concepts of evidence-based health care,

> 'Evidence based medicine is the conscientious, explicit and judicious use of current best evidence in making decisions about the care of individual patients' and 'evidence based medicine means integrating the individual clinical expertise with the best external clinical evidence from systematic research'.

However, their more recent definition also recognizes the significance of patient values in health care and defines evidence-based medicine as 'the integration of best research evidence with clinical expertise and patient values' (Sackett *et al.* 2004). These definitions indicate that it is a process driven by a way of thinking about patients or clients rather than a single intervention but also about the role of judgement as exercised by professionals' experience cognisant with patients' values. These same concepts can be seen in nursing definitions. DiCenso and Cullum (1998) in an editorial examining Evidence-based Nursing states 'Evidence-based nursing integrates the best evidence from research with clinical expertise, patient preferences, and existing resources into decision-making about the health care of individual patients' (DiCenso and Cullum 1998: 38). Note that in both definitions neither client choice nor professional expertise is lost in the pursuit of the goal of evidence-based practice. Importantly, both definitions signal the tentative nature of evidence. To practice evidence-based care, it is essential that you make judgements about what is 'best' evidence. Figure 10.1 clearly identifies the interrelatedness of these concepts.

Increasingly, you will find that the more generic terms 'evidence-based health care' and 'evidence-based practice' are now being used to characterize a process of identifying and evaluating knowledge in order to address practice-based questions. This terminology highlights the inter-professional nature of health care. You will find when accessing evidence for your practice that it can be derived from research undertaken by many professional groups and drawn from different theoretical disciplines. In the past Jordan (1997) suggested that in health care professions what has counted as 'valuable knowledge' and been passed on to other practitioners and clients is often determined by who holds power and status. The opinion of such authoritative experts can provide sources of knowledge but may not be adequate when used alone to inform complex decision-making. The store of an individual's experience is always growing and as such their opinion reflects an incomplete resource. The transmission of opinion alone leaves practitioners vulnerable to acceptance of outdated or unproven

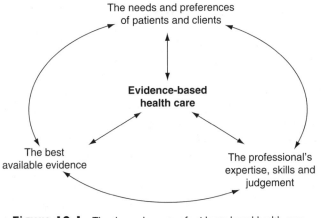

Figure 10.1   The three elements of evidence-based health care.
Source: CASP (2002: 12).

interventions. It may also engender reluctance to look at evidence that can be provided from other health care disciplines. Muir Gray (2001) suggests that the evidence-based movement is a shift from the reliance on opinion-based decision-making towards the acceptance and utilization of multiple forms of evidence. The challenge to practitioners like yourselves is to be able to access and appraise the sea of evidence that will confront you (see Chapter 11 which examines the critique and appraisal of evidence providing you with some frameworks for informing your judgements).

10.3 How does evidence-based practice relate to clinical effectiveness?

Decisions concerning health care must be driven by evidence of both cost and clinical effectiveness (National Health Service Executive [NHSE] 1996a). The goal of health care is to attain through the careful use of available resources the greatest possible improvement in the health of the United Kingdom population. Clinically effective care directly relates to the evidence-based health care. Clinical effectiveness is about taking forward evidence and applying it in practice. Clinically effective care achieves that which it claims to do in practice. The Royal College of Nursing succinctly describes this as 'doing the right thing in the right way, for the right patient, at the right time' (1996: 3). This means that in order to be clinically effective practitioners must base their practice on evidence and through clinical governance processes such as audit; this evidence must be shown to work (see Chapter 8). Accompanying any attempt to practise evidence-based health care must be an ongoing evaluation.

The mandate for cost-effective care led to concerns that the evidence-based movement was solely directed at saving money and could compromise the quality of individual care. It was thought that the standardization of care which evidence-based practice promotes may lead to the slavish following of 'cook book' approaches (DiCenso and Cullum 1998, Colyer and Kamath 1999). Indeed, evidence-based practice has been described as both 'arrogant and seductive' (Muir Gray 2001: 9). In using these terms, Muir Gray was advising caution about the unquestioning acceptance of some forms of evidence without careful consideration of the context to which that evidence is to be applied. In the early stages of evidence-based medicine, the evidence base for change was frequently derived from epidemiological studies (studies which study disease in groups of patients or populations). One criticism of this approach was that by focusing on populations rather than on individuals the delivery of individualized holistic care could be compromised. Whilst few practitioners would disagree about basing care on information about what works there still remains debate about what evidence *is* and what constitutes *best* evidence. It must be remembered that practitioners are working within a climate of increasing consumerism and choice. In Nursing and Midwifery, for example, this personal choice and individual focus is highlighted within the professional code as being key values of the profession (NMC 2004). All of these factors must be acknowledged when pursuing evidence-based health care. It needs to be recognized that there are two targets in the delivery of evidence-based health care. At the microlevel it is used to inform and enhance the care of individuals. At the macrolevel evidence-based decisions can be used for making wider public health policy decisions. Both elements will impact on the work of the individual practitioner. Colyer and Kamath (1999), in their review of the Evidence-Based Practice movement, argue that there is considerable congruence between government and professional perspectives.

ACTIVITY 10.1

Can you see any matches between the Code of Conduct statements for your professional group and the purposes of evidence-based practice as outlined in this chapter so far?

10.4 Benefits of evidence-based practice: Review of the factors leading to the evidence-based practice movement

Having defined evidence-based healthcare and its relationship to clinical effectiveness, this section of the chapter will address the intended benefits of the use of this process within health care. Proponents of evidence-based practice suggest that this approach safeguards against the use of practice which is ineffective and inefficient. The proviso is added that 'good' practitioners must use the evidence together with their own subjective interpretation of their client's situation. In this way professional expertise can be used to accommodate the clients' preferences and rights within the decision-making process. Without this component practice may become shaped by irrelevant or inapplicable evidence. Evidence-based practice can then be seen to incorporate both subjective and objective components into a clear decision-making process (CASP 2002, Hewitt-Taylor 2002).

By providing clinically effective health care within the constraints of available resources, evidence-based practice makes explicit the central and guiding principles of contemporary health care. Chapter 7 has already sensitized you to the need to secure particular goals in health care delivery. Goals such as quality, value for money and fitness for purpose can be used as indicators to determine the best evidence for health care decisions. The evidence-based practice initiative needs to be recognized as a way of securing the goals of general management and those which have led to the creation of the NHS internal market (Colyer and Kamath 1999, NHSE 1996a,b).

Evidence-based practice should move health care beyond opinion-led care to care which has an explicit evidence base. Combining this approach with the concept of clinical effectiveness further adds confidence in that the care proposed has been tried and tested. Importantly, by sharing with clients the rationales for their care there are discernible benefits. Early research has identified that clients who receive care based on research made gains in their knowledge about their condition in comparison to those receiving routinised care (Heater *et al.* 1988). Evidence-based practice is a key component within the development of National

Service Frameworks in which clients and carers will be given information about what they can expect from the health service.

ACTIVITY 10.2

As you read this chapter you may find it helpful to assemble a list of benefits and potential drawbacks of evidence-based practice. Do use your own experience in clinical practice to supplement what you have read.

10.5   Research and evidence-based practice

Since the previous definitions of evidence-based practice included the term 'research' it may be helpful at this point to consider what research is. Then the relationship of research to evidence-based practice can be clarified. An initial activity is provided in order for you to consider your position in some of the debates that relate to the place of research in evidence-based health care.

ACTIVITY 10.3

What does research mean to you?
What are the outcomes of research?
Who does it?
How do they do it?

Research includes thought and action processes. In its broadest form, it can include the reading and independent study that you undertake to develop an assignment or to examine a significant incident from your practice placements. More formally research is systematic enquiry conducted with the purpose of generating knowledge and may be undertaken by a designated researcher or a research team. Parahoo (1997: 10) suggests that it is the following of 'a system-atic process which leads to both data analysis and collection that differenti-ates research as a specific form of inquiry from more general attempts to find out something about something'. Therefore, considering research as a care-fully designed formal activity will be the starting point for the discussion which follows.

Before looking at the specific contribution of research to Evidence-Based Prac-tice, there are some essential differences between 'research' and 'evidence-based practice' which are often unrecognized and this leads to the two terms being used synonymously (Carnwell 2001). Although, both research and evidence-based practice are systematic processes each has a different purpose. Research is used to conduct an investigation the results of which will be used to add to existing evidence. Evidence-based practice on the other hand aims to search for and critically appraise evidence, some of which will be provided by research. Both research and evidence-based practice have differing endpoints which also provide a useful distinction between the two. Research ends with the outcomes specified at the start of the study which are then used to provide recommendations for further practice and research. Evidence-based practice ends with the making of clinical decisions which may involve a practice change in the light of the evidence. Research then is about gaining new knowledge but evidence-based practice as the name implies has its roots in practice and draws on research together with other evidence to bring about practice changes.

10.6 Research definitions and paradigms

'Research is not owned by any one profession or discipline, it is a systematic way of thinking and knowing and has a distinct vocabulary that can be learned and used by anyone' (De Poy and Giltin 1998: 5). This definition is particularly helpful as the work of health care professionals will be informed by an eclectic evidence base and will, for example, draw upon research in life sciences (anatomy and physiology) and social sciences (psychology, sociology). In contrast, a definition provided some 30 years ago stated 'research was a systematic controlled, empirical and critical investigation of natural phenomena guided by theory and hypotheses about the presumed relations amongst such phenomena' (Kerlinger 1986: 3). This second complex and restrictive definition suggests that there is one purpose and one way of doing research – to search for cause and effect. Kerlinger proposed that in order to achieve this aim controlled investigations were to be undertaken in the form of experiments. For many years these powerful ideas were shared by opinion leaders in medicine and health care. The widespread acceptance of this approach led to the use of a shorter term the 'scientific method' being used when talking of the (then) accepted ways to undertake research (Carter 1998). However, such a narrow definition of research does not capture all the questions that practitioners ask about the care they deliver or ways to find answers to those questions.

There is often heated debate about the best ways to answer health care questions when using research. Different research perspectives call in to question how human beings come to 'know' and understand their world. Philosophy directly relates to this as it is defined as 'the love, study, or pursuit of wisdom, or of knowledge of things and their causes, whether theoretical or practical' (Oxford English Dictionary 2004: 688). This *study* involves human reasoning and the use of specified systems of thought on these matters. The dictionary definition further states that this informs a 'general view or outlook' on life. In daily conversation we may have heard others saying my philosophy is . . . and in Chapters 1 and 2 you were asked to consider your values and philosophy in relation to nursing.

In health care, groups of practitioners come to have allegiance with particular philosophies and this influences their view of research. This is just as in everyday life individuals have different views on say parenting or marriage and this in turn shapes how they think and act. Importantly, with regard to the generation of evidence for health care the influence of particular forms of philosophical thought has literally shaped both what has been considered worthy of examination and the ways in which that examination will be done. This determines what questions about health care have been considered worthwhile and the ways in which answers to those questions have been accessed through research.

A very important philosophical concept is that of paradigms; they are cognitive structures (ways of thinking) which assist in the exploration of the events and experiences which constitute human life. Put more simply, a paradigm is a representation of how we see the world. A paradigm (and there are several) can most readily be considered as a particular lens through which we view and make sense of our daily experiences. Taking the lens analogy further, different lenses perhaps of differing colours or resolution would radically change what is viewed by the wearer. There is a relationship between the underpinning philosophical ideas, the paradigm, the methodology and methods employed to generate evidence. Acknowledging fundamental beliefs and values and understanding how these determine how research is conducted is a fundamental component of designing a research study. This section of the chapter will also show how this will shape the way in which you ask health care questions and influence the type of evidence that may answer your questions. To make this all clearer, two paradigms or perspectives will be considered together with their impact on evidence-based health care. The philosophical ideas underpinning each will be outlined and then linked to the types of questions asked and ways in which the answer might be derived.

The first research paradigm to be considered is that of positivism. This paradigm was supported by authoritative figures in the early nineteenth century and underpins the previously mentioned 'scientific method' (Goding and Edwards 2002). Positivism is based on the belief that knowledge is objective and that rules and causation can be discovered through the use of experimentation or direct observation. The researcher undertaking a study informed by positivism (in the positivistic tradition) would be engaged in measuring and determining relationships. Correspondingly the information (or data) produced by such research would be quantitative. It is this type of research you may have heard being described as 'quantitative research' which is to an extent a misnomer as it is the data produced which is being used to name the approach. However, this terminology has greater everyday familiarity than the term 'positivism'. Its use may help to convey something of the characteristics and aims of the research and it has become a short cut when talking about research that has as its aim objective measurement or description.

In contrast to positivism, the second paradigm, the interpretative or naturalistic paradigm, is founded on the belief that individual knowledge of the world is gained from a personal point of view and is context-specific. Professionals working within this paradigm are concerned with the meanings and understandings of the clients with whom they work rather than cause and effect. In contrast to the positivistic perspective, if a researcher was influenced by the values of the naturalistic paradigm, the study aims and design would be very different. The researcher would be exploring people's subjective experience without controlling

how they relate their experience or how they act. The researcher would be t
or observing people to better understand their world and gain insights. The
research would gain qualitative information about the subjective experiences of
individuals. This is sometimes called qualitative research or research which takes
a qualitative approach.

Carter (1998) suggests that research and the scientific method have been
used interchangeably and that this is unwise. The notion of *the* scientific method
immediately conjures up pictures of the laboratory, the experiment in other
words of an approach informed by positivism. Practitioners are able and indeed
required to use both perspectives in order to research health care. No one
perspective (paradigm) can provide the answers to all the questions. Different
paradigms must be respected and valued. The following activity has been
designed to show the value of research framed by the philosophical principles
underpinning both paradigms.

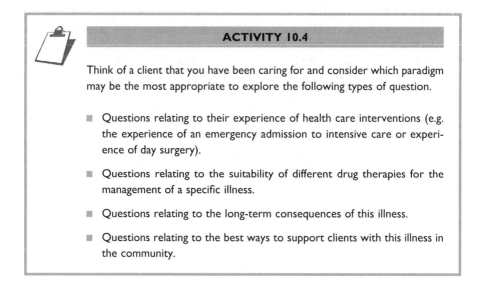

ACTIVITY 10.4

Think of a client that you have been caring for and consider which paradigm
may be the most appropriate to explore the following types of question.

- Questions relating to their experience of health care interventions (e.g.
  the experience of an emergency admission to intensive care or experience of day surgery).

- Questions relating to the suitability of different drug therapies for the
  management of a specific illness.

- Questions relating to the long-term consequences of this illness.

- Questions relating to the best ways to support clients with this illness in
  the community.

Caring interventions are multifaceted and embrace activities which are more
readily described as human encounters rather than interventions. For example,
you may have heard of the therapeutic relationship as a valuable part of caring
practices (see Chapter 2). Consider if this could or should ever be standardized
and measured? Critics of the evidence-based movement argue that if reliance is
placed on obtaining evidence on aspects of care that can be readily examined
and observed within positivistic research then it may oversimplify the realities of
practice and undervalue the interpersonal dimensions of caring.

It is important that you appreciate both of the paradigms are important in
providing evidence on which to base practice and can be combined in order
to gain the fullest possible picture. Regrettably, in the past there has been
a tendency for 'tribalism'– supporting one perspective over another without
critical consideration of what each may offer. More recently there has been

growing recognition of a diverse and exciting range of methods capable of addressing both the processes and the outcomes of health care (Pope and Mays 2002).

10.7 Research and hierarchies of evidence

When supporters of Evidence-Based Medicine, which was the 'parent' of Evidence-Based Practice, attempted to specify the type of evidence used to guide practice, considerable emphasis was placed on research and quantitative methods (Gilgun 2005). There was a common assumption that 'the' evidence was research evidence. To transmit this concept clearly and concisely 'evidence' was ordered within a hierarchy and each was ranked to show its superiority. The randomized controlled trial was seen as the gold standard of research. The randomized controlled trial is a form of experimental study yielding quantitative data and which is carefully designed to minimize the operation of chance and bias (Goding and Edwards 2002). In such hierarchies qualitative, non-controlled studies, which are sometimes criticized for being too subjective and difficult to interpret were placed at a lower ranking. Both quantitative and qualitative approaches were ranked above expert opinion which was placed at the lowest level. Later, systematic reviews (a review of a series of trials) became recognized within accepted hierarchies of evidence (Greenhalgh 2003, see Figure 10.2).

This idea of a hierarchy does however raise important questions for practitioners. How appropriate and accessible are these evidence forms for deciding what to do when faced with complex human situations and environments? For example, when resources are compromised and when there are tensions between the 'best possible' and the 'best available evidence'. Before discussing these

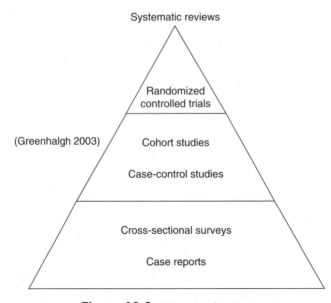

Figure 10.2 Hierarchy of evidence.
Source: Greenhalgh 2003.
Reproduced with permission from Blackwell Publishing.

points further you may find it helpful to consider your world of practice by undertaking the next activity.

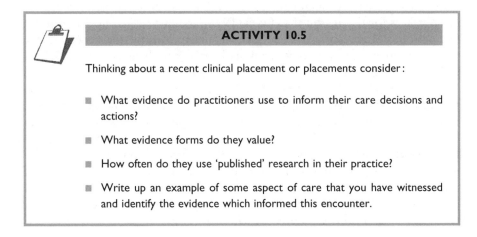

ACTIVITY 10.5

Thinking about a recent clinical placement or placements consider:

■ What evidence do practitioners use to inform their care decisions and actions?

■ What evidence forms do they value?

■ How often do they use 'published' research in their practice?

■ Write up an example of some aspect of care that you have witnessed and identify the evidence which informed this encounter.

10.8 Balancing clients' needs with available evidence

You may have identified that practitioners use a wider range of evidence than that within the hierarchy presented previously. In 1998, Mulhall noted that only a moderate proportion of nurses use research as a basis for practice. Part of the difficulty is thought to be that although nurses perceive research positively, they either cannot access the information or cannot judge the value of the studies which they find (see Chapter 12). Perhaps, more controversially, other authors suggest that it is not the inaccessibility of research but its irrelevance to individual unique caring encounters which is the source of the problem (Gilgun 2005, Rolfe and Gardner 2005). Le May (1999) suggests that the greater part of practitioners evidence resource draws upon experience and expert opinion. An alternative hierarchy has been proposed by Le May (1999) which shows research (all forms) as being the tip of the iceberg whose greater mass is comprised of experience, theory, evidence from clients and or carers, evidence from role models and experts and, finally, from policy directives. Colyer and Kamath (1999) affirm that good practitioners must synthesize both clinical expertise and the best available external evidence recognizing neither will suffice alone.

Judgements are required to determine which evidence sources are to be used and given primacy in hierarchies of evidence. For example, it may not be ethical to conduct experimental (positivistic) research on vulnerable clients such as children, clients who have mental health problems or those who have learning disabilities (Gates and Atherton 2001, Oliver *et al.* 2003). Additionally, even if results are available perhaps from a clinical trial on the efficacy, for example, of a type of antidepressant the practitioners may have difficulty in applying the results to the care of a specific client. The participants in trials are selected so that they do not have confounding variables (other factors that would detract from the effects of the intervention being examined). Depending on the study, 'unwanted' variables could include other illnesses, non-compliance or perhaps being obese. In real life the uniqueness of each individual means that there are variables which we cannot readily control and sometimes even struggle to identify. It is for this reason that Rolfe (1998) argues that it is not appropriate in a person-centred caring practice such as nursing to apply the general to the specific. There must be a place for clinical expertise, the client's needs and wishes and clinical judgement.

The debate about hierarchies can be futile in further generating dissention between widely different groups of health care practitioners who have differing views on the nature of evidence itself. Rycroft-Malone *et al.* (2004) suggest that by focusing on understanding and generating research evidence, the Evidence-Based Practice movement has failed to place emphasis on gaining a better understanding of the other forms of evidence that can be used in health care. They suggest that in order to practice person-centred evidence-based care what is required is acknowledging, accessing and using the widest evidence base for practice. In the process illustrated in Figure 10.3, it is important to recognize the potential of reflective practice to be placed at the heart of this process (see Chapters 3, 4 and 6) enabling practitioners to generate knowledge directly from and during their caring encounters with individuals (Rolfe and Gardner 2005).

In order to achieve this synthesis each practitioner is required to constantly ask questions about practice, building their own evidence base of what works in practice and then using this to compliment other evidence sources.

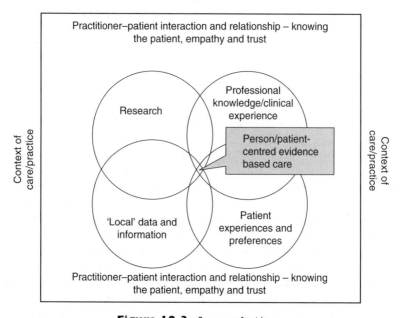

Figure 10.3 Sources of evidence.
Source: Rycroft-Malone *et al.* 2004.
Reproduced with permission from Blackwell Publishing.

10.9 Evidence-based health care starts with asking questions

> When in doubt, observe and ask questions. When certain, observe at length and ask many more questions.
>
> (General Patton 1947: 22)

This final section of the chapter considers how you can use the principles of evidence-based practice in your day-to-day caring for clients. Abbott *et al.* (2002) argue stronger emphasis should rest upon how well research (or indeed any evidence) answers the question rather than debating the merits of the approach adopted. Therefore, the asking of questions is central to evidence-based care and for those questions to capture the complexities of professional practice and be relevant to practice they must arise from practice itself. In a recent study examining the extent to which evidence-based practice could be implemented in one hospital trust, one factor restricting this change was the inability of practitioners in both framing questions and accessing evidence (Newman *et al.* 2000). It can be seen from Figure 10.4 that these elements are fundamental to the process of Evidence-Based Practice.

Questions relating to the care of individual clients need to be converted into answerable questions. The most frequently asked questions arising in clinical practice are those questions prefaced with *why do we do it this way? Or what would happen if?* If you wished to use the library resources to access evidence you would need to convert these thoughts into a search strategy. Framing the question in a way which lends itself to searching whilst still capturing the need of the particular client or service focus is an important stage to get right (Flemming 1998). This is not as easy as it sounds, as questions can be framed or set in a variety of different ways and the selection of individual words really counts. In fact, the words used will 'shape' what evidence is likely to be found in the second

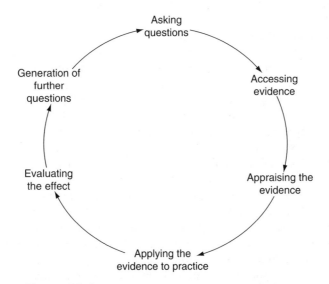

Figure 10.4 The cyclical process of Evidence-Based practice.

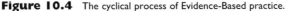

stage of the process. Exponents of the evidence-based medicine movement were the first to address the need for specificity in asking the question. They suggested the use of the 'PICO' format (Centre for Evidence Based Medicine 2005) which splits the question into four elements. Box 10.1 provides an explanation of 'PICO' with examples.

BOX 10.1 PICO = **P**opulation, **I**ntervention, **C**omparison, **O**utcome

Population   = Children in the first year of life
Intervention = Who have had bronchiolitis (an acute viral respiratory infection)
Comparison = Compared to children who have not had bronchiolitis
Outcome   = Likelihood of developing asthma

. . . so the question in full asks 'do children in the first year of life who have had bronchiolitis have a greater likelihood of the later development of asthma when compared to those children who have not had bronchiolitis'.

Source: Centre for Evidence Based Medicine (2005).

The benefits of using such an approach are in making clear identification of terms that may be used later for either free text or MeSH (Medical Subject Headings) terms searching for the evidence (see Chapter 11 and Jones and Smyth [2002] who provide a useful overview of this process). This type of specific question is considered to be more answerable as the boundaries for the process are set and it is clear, for example, which children are to be included (and conversely excluded) from your searches.

The downside is that considerable knowledge may be needed to frame the question in the first place. Additionally, some questions (as you have seen in Activity 10.4) relate to the experiences or perceptions of clients of health care rather than cause and effect. The notion of writing a question in the terms used within Figure 10.4 immediately presents some assumptions. For example, an outcome has to be specified in advance. By specifying an outcome in a possible relationship between events the PICO format generates a hypothesis. This is a statement that can be proved or disproved. If you recall the earlier discussion of paradigms you may remember that this 'proving' approach is in harmony with the intentions of research in the positivistic tradition. There is nothing the matter with asking this type of question, it is very valuable in some circumstances. In the example above, the answer would enable the nurse to predict which children may be more likely to develop asthma and this knowledge could be used to provide parental information. However, if you were more interested in what is it *like* to have a child admitted to hospital with breathing problems in the first year of life, this approach is too restrictive. A much more open-ended question without comparison literally gives space to explore widely and to discover rather than prove something. The process of finding evidence about a subjective experience (parent's views) becomes philosophically muddled if it is decided in advance what you are looking for by specifying outcomes and relationships. Here, it may be more useful to define the population and consider the intervention as an experience or process in which you are interested rather than an outcome. For example, you may be interested in perception. See Box 10.2 for an example of a question which uses a qualitative approach to its investigation.

BOX 10.2 PI(E)O Population, Intervention/Experience, Outcome

Population = Parents
Intervention or experience = Hospitalized child
Outcome = Parental perceptions

No comparison is required as the purpose is to gain in-depth information about subjective experiences. It is again possible to use such terms for searching and by combining their use you will be able to access evidence.

ACTIVITY 10.6

Thinking of your field of practice, develop three questions about the care of clients.
How easy is it to use the PICO format?
Does it limit the type of questions asked?
Does using this format focus only on some of the aspects of the care that you deliver?

10.10 Conclusion

This chapter has examined the development of Evidence-Based Practice and clarified its relationship to clinical effectiveness and research. In underlining the influence of two different research paradigms, I have emphasized the contribution that each can make to evidence-based practice and indicated why the unquestioning acceptance of either paradigm as having superiority over the other may undermine the potential of both to inform your practice. It has also emphasized how important it is to ensure that in embracing the concept of EBP we do not fail to lose sight of the central purpose of caring and the values that underpin that role. I have indicated that there are many tensions in determining what the 'best evidence' is to base practice on. Practitioners are very often challenged to examine the best available evidence rather than the best possible evidence and this will require considerable skill and judgement. The quest of EBP is to influence practice and that starts with the asking of clinical questions in your clinical practice. The next part of the 'journey' then is over to you . . .

=== **SELF-EVALUATION** ===

And, finally, your chance to revise what you have learnt from this chapter

- What is Evidence-Based Practice?

- What is Clinical Effectiveness?

- What is the connection between Evidence-Based Practice and Clinical Effectiveness?

- What is the difference between Evidence-Based Practice and Research?

- What is a research paradigm and how does it influence the way in which research is undertaken?

- What is a hierarchy of evidence?

- What has traditionally be placed at the top of a hierarchy of evidence?

- List four different forms of evidence?

- How many stages are there in the evidence-based process and what are they?

- What four 'ingredients' can be used in framing a question?

References

Abbott, P., McSherry, R., and Simmons, M. (2002) *Evidence-Informed Nursing: A Guide for Clinical Nurses.* Routledge, London.

Carnwell, R. (2001) Essential differences between research and evidence based practice. *Nurse Researcher* 8(2): 55–68.

Carter, B. (1998) *Perspectives on Pain Mapping the Territory.* Arnold, London.

Centre for Evidence Based Medicine (CEBM) (2005) *Focusing Clinical Questions.* CEBM, Oxford. http://www.cebm.net/focus_quest.asp [accessed online 15 June 2006].

Colyer, H. and Kamath, P. (1999) Evidence-based practice. A philosophical and political analysis: Some matters for consideration by professional practitioners. *Journal of Advanced Nursing* 29(1): 188–193.

Critical Appraisal Skills Programme (CASP) (2002) *Evidence Based Healthcare: An Open Learning Resource for Health Care Practitioners.* CASP, Oxford.

De Poy, E. and Giltin, L.N. (1998) *Introduction to Research: Understanding and Applying Multiple Strategies* (Second edition). Mosby, St Louis.

DiCenso, A. and Cullum, N. (1998) Implementing evidence based nursing: Some misconceptions. *Evidence Based Nursing* 1: 38–39.

Flemming, K. (1998) Asking answerable questions. *Evidence Based Nursing* 1: 36–37.

Gates, B. and Atherton, H. (2001) Learning disability nursing. The challenge of evidence based practice for learning disabilities. *British Journal of Nursing* 10(8): 517–522.

Gilgun, F. (2005) The four cornerstones of evidence based social work. *Research on Social Work Practice* 15(1): 52–61.

Goding, L. and Edwards, K. (2002) Evidence-based practise. *Nurse Researcher* 9(4): 45–57.

Greenhalgh, T. (2003) *How to Read a Paper: The Basics of Evidence Based Medicine.* BMJ Publishing Group, London.

Heater, B.S., Becker, A.M., and Olson, R.K. (1988) Nursing interventions and patient outcomes: A meta-analysis of studies. *Nursing Research* 37(5): 303–307.

Hewitt-Taylor, J. (2002) Evidence based practice. *Nursing Standard* 17: 14–15, 47–52.

Jones, L.V. and Smyth, R.L. (2002) How to perform a literature search. *Current Paediatrics* 12: 138–143.

Jordan, B. (1997) Authoritative knowledge and its construction. In: Davis-Floyd, R.E. and Sargent, F. (1997) (eds) *Childbirth and Authoritative Knowledge: Cross Cultural Perspectives.* University of California Press, Berkeley.

Kerlinger, K. (1986) *Foundations of Behavioural Research* (Third edition). Holt Rinehart and Winston, London.

Le May, A. (1999) *Evidence-Based Practice.* Nursing Times Clinical Monographs No 1. NT Books, London.

Muir Gray, J.A. (2001) *Evidence-Based Healthcare.* Churchill Livingstone, Edinburgh.

Mulhall, A. (1998) Nursing, research and the evidence. *Evidence Based Nursing* 1: 4–6.

National Health Service Executive (NHSE) (1996a) *Promoting Clinical Effectiveness: A Framework for Action in and through the NHS.* NHSE, Leeds.

National Health Service Executive (NHSE) (1996b) *Clinical Guidelines: Using Clinical Guidelines to Improve Patient Care within the NHS.* NHSE, Leeds.

Newman, M., Papadopoulos, I. and Melifonwu, R. (2000) Developing organizational systems and culture to support evidence-based practice: The experience of the Evidence-Based Ward Project. *Evidence-Based Nursing* 3: 103–104.

Nursing Midwifery Council (NMC) (2004) *The NMC Code of Professional Conduct: Standards for Conduct, Performance and Ethics.* NMC, London.

Oliver, P.C., Piachaud, J., Done, J., Regan, A., Cooray, S.E., and Tyrer, P. (2003) Difficulties in developing evidence based approaches in learning disabilities. *Evidence-Based Mental Health* 6: 37–39.

Oxford English Dictionary (1989) *The Oxford English Dictionary* (Second edition) (Prepared Simpson, J. and Weiner, E.). Clarendon Press, Oxford.

Parahoo, K. (1997) *Nursing Research: Principles, Process and Issues.* Palgrave, Basingstoke.

Patton, G.S. Jr. (1947) *War As I Knew It.* (Annotated by Harkins, P.S.). Houghton Mifflin, Boston.

Pope, C. and Mays, N. (2002) *Qualitative Research in Healthcare* (Second edition). British Medical Journal, London.

Rolfe, G. (1998) The theory–practice gap in nursing: From research based practice to practitioner based research. *Journal of Advanced Nursing* 28(3): 672–679.

Rolfe, G. and Gardner, L. (2005) Towards a nursing science of the unique evidence, reflexivity and the study of persons. *Journal of Research in Nursing* 10(3): 297–310.

Royal College of Nursing (RCN) (1996) *Clinical Effectiveness Royal College of Nursing Guide.* RCN, London.

Rycroft-Malone, J., Seers, K., Titchen, A., Harvey, G., Kitson, A., and McCormack, B. (2004) What counts as evidence in evidence-based practice? *Journal of Advanced Nursing* 47(1): 81–90.

Sackett, D., Rosenberg, W., Gray, J.A.M., Haynes, R.B., and Richardson, W.S. (1996) Evidence based medicine: What it is and what it isn't. *British Medical Journal* 312: 71–72.

Sackett, D., Strauss, S., Richardson, W., Rosenberg, W., and Haynes, R. (2004) *Evidence Based Medicine: How to Practice and Teach EBM.* Churchill Livingstone, London.

@ Useful resources to explore evidence-based practice and research

Websites worth visiting

http://ebn.bmjjournals.com/
Evidence Based Nursing online which is accessible without a subscription if you already subscribe to one of the Nursing Standard group of journals such as *Nurse Researcher* or *Nursing Standard.*

http://ebn.bmjjournals.com/misc/previous.shtml
Editors in Evidence Based Nursing 'choices' which are free to all visitors and are helpful in giving those new to research examples of different research designs.

http://bmjupdates.mcmasetr.ca/index.asp
A searchable database provided by the BMJ publishing group and McMaster University Health Information Research Unit which aims to provide access to current best evidence tailored to individual health care interests to support evidence-based clinical decisions. Citations from over 110 journals are pre-rated for quality by research staff and practising physicians. Accessing this resource provides a searchable database of medical literature and links to selected evidence-based resources.

http://www.tripdatabase.com/index.cfm
TRIP was created in 1997 to bring together all the evidence-based health care resources available on the Internet. It started with 1100 links recorded from 15 sources and since then it has grown rapidly in both coverage and usability. This expansion has also encompassed the addition of new forms of material including peer-reviewed journals and etextbooks. This is a subscription site but the first five searches are free and it may be useful to have a look under a topic of interest to see the range of evidence sources which will be identified from patient information leaflets to clinical guidelines and primary research.

http://www.cebm.net/toolbox.asp
The 'toolbox' is an assortment of materials which are very useful for practitioners. Although housed at the Centre for Evidence Based Medicine, Oxford site, the information relating to asking questions, types and levels of evidence and advantages and disadvantages of different study types, is applicable to all groups of health care professionals.

Suggested reading

Abbott, P., McSherry, R., and Simmons, M. (2002) *Evidence-Informed Nursing: A Guide for Clinical Nurses.* Routledge, London.
A very useful introductory guide for nurses and other health care professionals. The requirement for evidence-based practice is examined together with an exploration of how evidence should be used in the clinical setting.

Carnwell, R. (2001) Essential differences between research and evidence based practice. *Nurse Researcher* 8(2): 55–68.
This paper clarifies the differences between research and evidence-based practice. Carnwell explores how evidence-based practice can complement the findings from research by ensuring that valid and relevant research is used to inform clinical decision-making.

Flemming, K. (1998) Asking answerable questions. *Evidence Based Nursing* 1: 36–37.
A short and very readable introductory paper that summarizes the process of evidence-based nursing and gives helpful tips for asking questions in a way which will enhance searching for evidence.

Rycroft-Malone, J., Seers, K., Titchen, A., Harvey, G., Kitson, A., and McCormack, B. (2004) What counts as evidence in evidence-based practice? *Journal of Advanced Nursing* 47(1): 81–90.
A thorough review of evidence-based practice within the context of contemporary health care. A paper that is comprehensive in examining the issues that arise from the quest for evidence-based care.

11

Critique and Appraisal of Evidence

Paula Libberton and Janice Brown

CONTENTS

- Searching the literature

- Critical thinking

- Concept of appraisal

- Purpose of appraisal

- Critical appraisal skills

- Appraisal tools and frameworks

LEARNING OUTCOMES

This chapter should enable you to

- Search the literature

- Appreciate the concept and practice skills of critical thinking

- Understand the concept of appraisal in relation to evidence-based practice

- Appreciate the purpose of appraisal in providing evidence-based care

- Develop your skills to appraise different forms of evidence

- Discuss the variety of frameworks available to assist in the process of appraisal

11.1 Introduction

The aim of this chapter is to introduce you to the concepts and skills necessary to search for evidence, to critique and appraise evidence in response to questions you have generated from practice. The purpose of the chapter is to support you in understanding and applying these concepts and skills in pursuit of becoming competent in evidence-based practice. Box 11.1 recaps the five steps in the evidence-based practice process. Step one, asking the question, has already been considered in Chapter 10.

BOX 11.1 Steps in the evidence-based practice process

Step one: Decide what you want to find out and construct a clear question to **ask**

Step two: **Find** the evidence which answers your question

Step three: **Appraise** the evidence you have found to see if it is valid and useful

Step four: **Act** on what you have found by applying it in practice, if appropriate

Step five: **Evaluate** the impact of this evidence on your practice

Source: Adapted from The Critical Appraisal Skills Programme (2002).

At the end of the chapter you will find suggested reading which is an important supplement to the ideas introduced here. It is particularly advisable to become aware of research texts which will provide you with information about specific aspects of research essential for effectively appraising research studies.

11.2 Searching for evidence

When faced with securing evidence to find responses to your carefully considered practice-based question, it is unsurprising that the beginning may feel over-whelming. Not only do you have to consider the types of evidence that may be suitable but also where and how to find it. A strategic approach (see Box 11.2) to finding and dealing with evidence can help with this process. However, do remember to draw on the resources and skills of your discipline-specific librarian, where available. Much of your search for evidence will probably revolve around published literature. In this light, it is amazing to think that over 2 million articles in 20,000 journals are published annually with over 400 journals specific to nursing (Thompson and Cullum 1999). Go to Activity 11.1 which may help you to begin searching the literature more effectively.

BOX 11.2 Stages of a literature search strategy

1. Develop your question/hypothesis

2. Write down all the keywords you can think of in relation to your question

3. Decide in advance types of evidence which would be most useful to respond to your question

4. Decide in advance where you are going to look, for example, electronic databases, index collections and experts

5. Do as broad a search as possible at first

6. Narrow your search by rejecting unhelpful materials (inclusion/exclusion criteria)

7. Review success and rework strategy if necessary (broaden or narrow)

Source: Adapted from Thompson (1999).

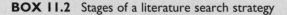

ACTIVITY 11.1

Identify your practice question or if you do not have one use the following to complete this activity:

'What are the most effective complementary interventions for helping asthma sufferers?'

1. Write down the initial keywords, for example asthma, complementary medicine, interventions

2. Identify the types of evidence that might be helpful: Intervention studies, cohort studies, qualitative studies

3. Consider which databases/sources might be most suitable, for example CINAHL, MEDLINE, Cochrane, experts, clinicians

4. Try searching the literature now to secure evidence for this question or a question of your own

11.3 Searching the literature

The principle of filtering is useful to remember, where you keep thinking and deciding on the most appropriate forms of evidence for your type of question. For example, if you have a question about effectiveness then looking for systematic reviews and randomized controlled trials would be helpful. MEDLINE,

Cochrane and CINAHL are examples of databases which may offer what you are looking for. If however you are more concerned with how people feel about certain treatments then survey and qualitative studies might be more useful to you. If you want to know what happens to people who have a specific disease then look for cohort studies. If you are interested in why some patients comply with treatments and others do not then qualitative studies and prospective cohort studies are useful. It really is a matter of understanding the methodological appropriateness of the types of evidence to support your question (see Chapter 10). The question posed normally guides the methodological stance that will be taken to discover the desired knowledge. An introductory understanding of types of knowledge and research design is therefore most helpful. If methodological issues are a concern to you then do refer to a research book that has been recommended on your programme.

In terms of pursing the literature search, as well as electronic databases, it is important to consider other sources. Searching by hand may feel time-consuming and unnecessary but it can help to cascade references from useful literature by looking at their reference sections. Communicating with experts, examining internal and external reports, reading dissertations (grey literature), scanning new journals and conference extracts are other useful sources.

You may feel at this stage that you are engaged to your computer and/or are living in the library. It takes time to search for evidence, so be patient and where possible go for the online versions but remember the cost involved in printing and photocopying. It can be frustrating if the library does not stock the journal you need or the particular issue number is not present. Interlibrary loans may be restricted in undergraduate courses so do use online journals where possible to secure your evidence. Once you have started to collect evidence, do not forget to read it and engage with it. Make notes and start a classification system to record its relevance – you could use a rating of 1 (interesting but not very relevant) to 5 (really relevant). Having a large pile of papers may feel comforting but will not answer your question on its own. At this stage, however, it is important to start making a list of criteria that will help you reject some of the literature as well as keeping some. This is called making inclusion and exclusion criteria and is stage 6 in a literature search (see Box 11.2). Activity 11.2 may help you develop your own inclusion/exclusion criteria.

ACTIVITY 11.2

If your practice question was:

'What are the most effective complementary interventions for helping asthma sufferers?'

What might your obvious inclusion and exclusion criteria be? Consider the following:

- Think about your target group, for example adults, children, older people.

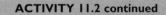

ACTIVITY 11.2 continued

- Think about the year/time frame when complementary therapies started to become popular.

- Think about the range of complementary therapies that are available.

Apply these principles to your own research question.

11.4 Purpose of critical appraisal

Assuming that you now have a good selection of evidence ranging from expert reports to published literature, your next question is how can I use the evidence I have? The main question that is useful to guide you here is: Is the evidence good enough to base my practice on? This leads us into consideration of critical appraisal. Appraisal is the third step of the evidence-based practice process (see Figure 11.1). The importance of this step is that once the evidence has been appraised, it might then be applied to practice. Without appraisal, the evidence-based practice process becomes invalid. It is not satisfactory to accept any evidence at face value without first checking out its truthfulness and applicability to the situation.

In order to consider the purpose of appraisal, it is essential to appreciate a definition of the term. Le May (1999) reinforces that it is a systematic process of deciding whether the evidence is good enough to base practice on. This process needs to provide a constructive review or criticism of the evidence to allow a judgement to be made about the value of the evidence in a specific context (Long 2002). The 'value' is in relation to the results/outcomes of the evidence as well as the methodological rigour or 'strength' of the evidence. It is unsafe to use the findings from a piece of evidence that is seriously flawed in its development or source.

Three elements are therefore important in conducting a critical appraisal: first are skills in critical thinking, second is the identification of the most appropriate tool to guide the critique and third is having an understanding of the type of evidence in question to know the rules of rigour agreed by the wider community.

11.5 Skills of critical thinking

Critical thinking takes time, patience and much practice, as it can be a highly complex activity. It can rely on self-awareness as well as technique, as it involves perseverance and practice. The more experience and knowledge we have in a relevant context the easier it is to practice critical thinking skills effectively. Critical thinking is about your judgement of the materials in question, where you need to decide on what is good and not so good, what is the value of the material and what is the potential for its application. Garratt *et al.* (2000) suggest there are four broad skills in critical thinking: analysing, making judgements, retrieving information and experimenting. These skills are synonymous with the characteristics of sound decision-making, both of which are essential components of practice and research. Case (1994) offers six characteristics of critical thinking (see Box 11.3) which can be a useful reflective tool.

BOX 11.3 Characteristics of critical thinking

1. Reframe the problem (or situation)

2. Seek input, share ideas and critique from others

3. Develop an attitude to inquiry

4. Have a sound knowledge base

5. Remember critical thinking is a skill and requires practice

6. It is beyond problem solving.

Source: Adapted from Case (1994).

Reframing the problem (or situation) means we need to consider other perspectives. This is probably one of the greatest challenges in critical thinking as we need to go beyond our own experiences and expand our perspectives by continually questioning ourselves and others who have differing perspectives. Questions that can be helpful here are: Is this an assumption or a fact? What evidence supports this inference? How closely does this inference support reality? How can I check out the validity for this conclusion? You might well have identified your initial practice question but, in the process of searching for and appraising the evidence, be prepared to modify and reframe your question. A common error in the evidence-based practice process is to base your findings on your initial thoughts rather than what your literature searching and appraisal have revealed.

Much can be gained from seeking input, sharing ideas and receiving critique from others. Multiple perspectives from multiple people may feel confusing at first but it can be used productively to develop your list of critical ideas. Living with uncertainty is not always a comfortable position to be in but it can also be viewed as a very exciting and liberating place in the context of critical thinking. An attitude to inquiry may not be natural but if the question 'Why?' is iterated enough times through practice, then it moves us to question our assumptions – our taken-for-granted world. It can be added to with other questions such as 'What else?' and 'What if?' Critical thinking manipulates facts and their known relationships to each other. The more knowledge you have, the more perspectives you will develop. This is why a sound knowledge base of the topic allows you greater scope to question assumptions. A sound knowledge base of methodological approaches used in the research literature and other types of evidence can also help if there are issues that you are unsure about.

ACTIVITY 11.3

Improve your knowledge of methodological approaches used in the research literature by reading them up in a research textbook. Perhaps start by finding out what a cohort study is or how grounded theory is defined.

Be patient and persevere in developing your critical thinking as it is a skill and requires practice. It will not just happen, so it is helpful to practice and to resist the urge to make hasty decisions. Finally, it is beyond problem solving, as there is the need to frame and reframe the problem. As you continue in your evaluation of the chosen solution (if there is one), reconsider alternatives you may have rejected initially. The attitude of enquiry demands generating, testing and assembling evidence to support a variety of solutions. Constructive criticism should involve identifying the strengths and weaknesses of a piece of evidence and provide ways in which these weaknesses could be overcome. It is essential to explain how and why the judgement was arrived at so that the process is made transparent to anyone who may question its truthfulness.

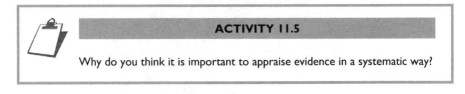

ACTIVITY 11.4

What is your attitude to enquiry?
What is your view on the model offered by Case (1994)?

11.6 Why bother with critical appraisal?

If we employed the skills of critical thinking to our evidence then we could pose the question of why bother with critical appraisal. We can be critical of evidence as it is presented without making a judgement as to its rigour. Indeed, to act on unreliable evidence is probably worse than acting without any evidence at all: to do so can at best destroy the values and practice of a profession, at worse it can cause harm to patients (CASP 2002). Therefore, critical appraisal is the process of systematically examining research evidence to assess its validity, results and relevance before using it to inform a decision (Hill and Spittlehouse 2003).

ACTIVITY 11.5

Why do you think it is important to appraise evidence in a systematic way?

We know that evidence comes in many forms, from systematic reviews of randomized controlled trials to personal experience of working with patients/clients with a particular condition (types of evidence was explored in Chapter 10). It is not only published research that requires appraisal but all evidence upon which we base clinical decisions about patient/client care. The questions that are asked in order to appraise a piece of evidence will depend on the type of evidence and the purpose for which it is required. However, what should be considered in all cases is: Whether the quality of the evidence is good enough to use the findings; what the results mean for the patients/clients; and whether the findings are applicable in the given setting (Newman and Roberts 2002), see Figure 11.1.

Health care professionals are increasingly being encouraged to use published literature in the form of research studies as a basis for their care practices (The interface between research and evidence-based practice is explored in Chapter 10.) It is vital that we have the skills to 'separate the wheat from the chaff' if we are going to do the right thing in the right way and at the right time to the right patient/client (Royal College of Nursing 1996).

The skills required to successfully appraise evidence may be seen by some as complex and out of reach. However, on one level we appraise everything that we read, as we automatically make a judgement as to whether the conclusion applies to our particular area of practice. The more practice we have in appraisal, the more questions we generate about our practice. This in turn increases the need for a systematic process of checking out the evidence. Initial questions to ask may be: Is there a clear decision trail leading to the results/outcomes? Can you trust the results/outcomes? What do the results mean? Are they relevant to your practice? The general rule is not to assume that any aspect of the research (or evidence) is sound!

ACTIVITY 11.6

Imagine that you are in a practice setting discussing the purpose of appraising evidence for practice. Can you think of any concerns that practitioners may have about working in this way? How could you assist them in seeing the benefits of evidence-based practice and the role that they have to play in making this a success?

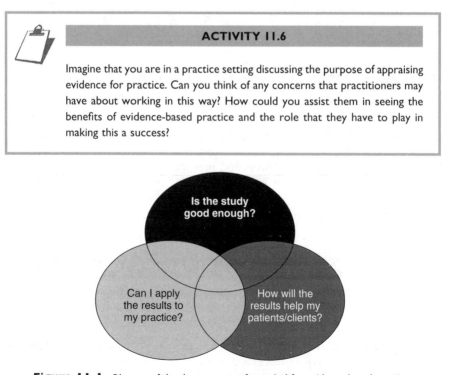

Figure 11.1 Diagram of the three aspects of appraisal for evidence-based practice.
Source: Adapted from Newman and Roberts (2002).

11.7 Starting the appraisal process

A good place to begin is to appraise published evidence in the form of journal articles. It is perhaps appropriate at this stage to consider what most of us do when we read a journal article. It is quite common for busy practitioners to just read the abstract. This may appear to provide an overview of the findings but if you read further you may find the reality to be quite different. Abstracts are written to entice the reader and are often very selective in their content. Therefore, it is very important to engage with the material in more detail in order to get the full picture.

ACTIVITY 11.7

Think about the last time you read a journal article. Did you read it in depth? If so, was the abstract a true reflection of the content of the article? Try reading another journal article and take particular note of what the abstract says in comparison to the journal article itself. Would you want someone to base your care just on the abstract?

11.8 Tools for appraising evidence

Now that you have begun to think about the journal article in some detail, it is useful to have a set of questions to guide your appraisal so it becomes systematic. The sort of questions you need to ask will depend on the type of article. Critical appraisal tools are available to help us in this activity (see Crombie 1996, DePoy and Giltin 1998, Greenlaugh 2001). These are checklists or frameworks with a series of questions that can lead to an informed judgement on the merits of the article and the meaning of the findings and their relevance.

In general terms, standard research appraisal questions can be divided into five sections which usually reflect the research process and mirror the structure of the article: introduction; methods; results; discussion; and conclusion. The introduction should give a clear indication of the rationale for the research along with the aims or better still a concise question. The methods section should provide information on how the study was conducted by giving details of the research design, sample, access, data collection, data analysis and ethical issues where appropriate. The results should be clearly presented in relation to the question. The discussion should offer an interpretation of the results, along with comments about the strengths and weaknesses of the study and further research required. Finally, the conclusion should report on any implications of the findings for future practice. See Box 11.4 for the kind of questions that can be asked to address each of the five sections.

BOX 11.4 Summary of questions to consider when reading a research study

Introduction:	What was the rationale for the research study?
	What were the aims of the study?
	What is the research question?
Methods:	How was the study carried out?
	What was the research design?
	How was the sample selected?
	How was the data collected?
	How was the data analysed?
	Were ethical issues considered?
Results:	Are these clearly presented?
	Do the results presented answer the research question?
Discussion:	Is an interpretation of the results offered?
	Are the strengths and weaknesses of the study analysed?
	Is further research suggested?
Conclusion:	Are the implications for future practice summarized?

Source: Adapted from Long (2002).

It is important to remember that critical appraisal is not about pulling a research study to pieces but is about identifying the limitations of the study (Bury and Jerosch-Herold 1998). In reality, there is no such thing as a perfect research study but that does not mean that we cannot learn from it. It is our responsibility when appraising a research study to decide whether the limitations of the study undermine the findings such that they cannot be applied to practice (Cutcliffe and Ward 2003). Therefore, we should be aiming to produce a more balanced and constructive review of the research study. This does not mean that we must identify the same number of strengths and weaknesses as this would create an artificial and somewhat valueless appraisal. Indeed, it is widely accepted that some research studies are of a higher quality than others and this should be reflected in the appraisal.

In addition to appraising component parts of the research study to make a judgement about its truthfulness, it is important to also think about whether the study can be applied to your patient/client and the setting within which you are practising. It is essential to consider the applicability of the study in this way, as this is the main reason for encouraging practitioners to learn the skills of appraisal. We want patients/clients to receive care based on the best available evidence which will ideally originate from a well-conducted research study (see Chapter 10 for a discussion of what constitutes good evidence). Appraisal skills are essential for making decisions about whether or not to change practice based on these studies (Cutcliffe and Ward 2003).

11.9 Frameworks for appraising research studies

The wide range of frameworks available for appraising research studies includes: Duffy's (1985) research appraisal checklist for evaluating nursing research; Burns and Grove's (1987) critical appraisal approach to critiquing nursing research; Morrison's (1991) approach to critiquing nursing research; and Polit and Hungler's (1997) approach to critiquing nursing research. Each framework has its advantages and disadvantages and these should be carefully considered before it is used. However, it is important to choose the correct type of critical appraisal tool to fit the evidence in hand.

Duffy's (1985) checklist produces a numerical value based on 51 criteria which is representative of the overall quality of the paper. It is orientated towards evaluating quantitative studies and may not be appropriate for appraising qualitative studies. Burns and Grove's (1987) appraisal tool consists of eight guidelines that the reviewer should be mindful of when asking a series of questions which are categorized under 11 key headings. The approach is easy to follow but like Duffy's (1985) approach its focus is on quantitative studies. Burns and Grove recognize that qualitative studies require a different set of appraisal questions to quantitative studies. As a result, they introduced a separate and comprehensive approach to appraising qualitative studies in the third edition (1997) of their book.

Morrison's (1991) approach to critiquing research outlines five central features along with questions that are categorized under seven headings. This approach is easy to follow and differs from the previous approaches in that it asks more open-ended questions which allow the reviewer to provide evidence to support their criticisms. It also encourages the reviewer to consider how the findings may impact on practice. However, as with Duffy's (1985) and Burns and Grove's (1987) approaches there is a focus on appraising quantitative studies.

Polit and Hungler (1997) offer a very thorough and comprehensive approach to appraising a study. They appear to have built upon previous approaches to create a framework which considers five key areas with varying numbers of questions under each heading. Polit and Hungler (1997) have a clear orientation for quantitative studies. Worked examples using these four frameworks can be found in a book edited by Cutcliffe and Ward (2003). Although the papers that they have chosen to appraise are related to mental health nursing, the principles will be the same for any area of practice. It is a good idea to read a worked example as this will show you how the framework can be effectively used and offer you the confidence to have a go yourself.

ACTIVITY 11.9

Now that you have tried using a simple set of questions (Box 11.4) to appraise a paper perhaps you may wish to start thinking about the paper in more detail. Find one of the appraisal tools discussed previously, or one of your own, and try using it to appraise a paper. Experiment until you find a framework that suits your needs.

11.10 Frameworks for appraising different forms of evidence

Evidence comes in many forms. So far we have considered appraisal frameworks for quantitative research studies. The frameworks that have been discussed have not differentiated between the different methodologies that are used to carry out research. Although it has been suggested that the approaches discussed were not really designed with qualitative research in mind. However, there is a need to have a specific tool to appraise a particular type of evidence. In order to know which framework to use, it is first necessary to identify the type of evidence. It may be simple to differentiate between clinical guidelines and a research study but it is not so easy to decide on the type of research if your research knowledge is limited. It is for this reason that it was suggested at the start of this chapter that there will be a need for you to become aware of research books to consult in such situations.

11.11 Appraising qualitative research

Qualitative research concentrates on people's experiences, attitudes and beliefs (Seers 2005). It is used to understand people's perceptions and consequently their actions (Boulton and Fitzpatrick 1997). It is concerned with the construction of meaning in social interactions (Popay and Williams 1998). Therefore, the framework used to appraise a qualitative study needs to reflect this research approach. The term 'qualitative research' like quantitative research covers a number of methodologies. Examples of qualitative approaches include: phenomenology; grounded theory; and ethnography. Explanations of each of these approaches can be found in most nursing research textbooks, for example Polit and Beck (2004).

The frameworks available to appraise studies that fall under the umbrella of qualitative research do not always distinguish between the different approaches. There are many sets of questions designed to assist in the appraisal process. A recent example is a framework by Spencer *et al.* (2003) which consists of 18 appraisal questions based on four central principles. These are that research should advance knowledge, be defensible in design, be rigorous in conduct and credible in claim. These questions can be accessed by visiting www.policyhub.gov.uk/evalpolicy/qual_eval.asp which is a Cabinet Office website. Another well-recognized framework for appraising qualitative research is available via the Critical Appraisal Skills Programme (CASP). This tool contains 10 questions to assist in the appraisal process. These questions cover three broad areas: rigour, credibility and relevance and were updated in 2002. This tool can be downloaded by visiting www.phru.nhs.uk/casp/qualitat.htm. CASP is part of the National Health Service and may therefore appeal more to health professionals than the tool provided by the National Centre for Social Research. Holloway and Wheeler (1996) offer tools for evaluating ethnography based on criteria established by Leininger (1994) and grounded theory based on the work of Strauss and Corbin (1990). You may find these tools useful if you have identified the methodology used in your research paper to be either ethnography or grounded theory.

ACTIVITY 11.10

Visit the CASP website (www.phru.nhs.uk/casp/qualitat.htm) and download the appraisal tool for qualitative research studies. Familiarize yourself with it. Look up any words that you do not understand. Try using it to appraise a paper of your choice that reports on a qualitative piece of research.

11.12 Appraising clinical guidelines

Clinical guidelines are somewhat different to the research studies that we have thought about appraising so far. Clinical guidelines are based on secondary evidence. They have the purpose of providing guidance by making recommendations which aim to improve health care and reduce unnecessary variations in care delivery (Snowball 2005). Therefore, they need to be based on the best available evidence, credible and well disseminated. Clinical guidelines can be broadly defined as systematically developed statements supporting decision-making and concerned with specific clinical problems (Hutchinson and Baker 1999). In the past many clinical guidelines have not been sufficiently based on the evidence (NHS Centre for Reviews and Dissemination 1994).

As with research studies, it is extremely important to appraise clinical guidelines to check that they are as accurate and useful as the purpose for which they were designed. There are a variety of frameworks available to assist in the appraisal of existing clinical guidelines and also the construction of new ones. The most up to date of these has been developed by the AGREE (Appraisal of Guidelines Research and Evaluation) Collaboration (2003). This instrument has been tested by researchers and guideline developers from 13 different countries

(Snowball 2005). It has been approved and recommended for use by the National Institute for Clinical Excellence (NICE) (www.nice.org.uk) who are responsible for producing national guidelines and technology appraisals in England and Wales and by the Scottish Intercollegiate Guidelines Network (SIGN) (www.sign.ac.uk) who are responsible for Scotland's guidelines.

The AGREE instrument consists of 24 statements under 7 headings. The headings are: (1) scope and purpose; (2) stakeholder involvement; (3) rigour of development; (4) clarity and presentation; (5) applicability; (6) editorial independence; and (7) overall assessment. The clinical guideline is appraised against each statement on a scale of 1 (strongly disagree) to 4 (strongly agree). There is supplementary information in the text of the instrument to assist in the appraisal process. The guideline itself is available from the AGREE Collaboration website (www.agreecollaboration.org).

ACTIVITY 11.11

Visit the AGREE Collaboration website (www.agreecollaboration.org) and download the AGREE instrument. Use the instrument to appraise a clinical guideline of your choice. You could choose either a local guideline or visit the NICE website (www.nice.org.uk) and select a national guideline which interests you.

11.13 Appraising systematic reviews

Another important form of evidence that is used to answer clinical questions is the systematic review. This is a secondary form of evidence which draws on primary research to answer a specific question. The Cochrane Library (2003) describes a systematic review as using systematic and explicit methods to select and critically appraise relevant research and to collect and analyse data from those studies to answer a clearly formulated question. The analysis and summary of the studies may or may not involve statistical methods (meta-analysis). It is expected that the review could be replicated by another person who would reach the same general conclusions if given access to the same resources (Dixon *et al.* 1997). Systematic reviews are popular with busy health care professionals who do not have the time to appraise all the available evidence themselves. However, it is essential that systematic reviews are appraised in the same way that other forms of evidence are before they are used to inform practice. There are a variety of frameworks available to assist in appraising systematic reviews. Most of these are in the form of checklists which focus on systematic reviews of randomized controlled trials with meta-analysis. This does not mean that systematic reviews of other forms of evidence are any less important. Accordingly, frameworks for appraising systematic reviews of other forms of evidence are in the process of being developed and made more readily available.

ACTIVITY 11.12

See if you can find a framework or checklist for appraising systematic reviews of other forms of evidence (not randomized controlled trials with meta-analysis). You might want to start by looking for a checklist for appraising a systematic review of qualitative research. Make a list of where you can access these checklists so that you have a list of resources available to you for future use.

The framework that will be presented here is one that was developed by Oxman *et al.* (1994). It is suggested that this is the most accessible framework for individuals who are appraising systematic reviews for the first time (Seers 2005). The framework is divided into three sections: (1) are the results valid? (2) if they

BOX 11.5 Questions to ask about systematic reviews

a) Are the results valid?

　　1. was a clear review question presented?

　　2. Were the right kind of studies used?

　　3. Was the search for studies thorough?

　　4. Were the studies critically appraised?

　　5. Did they explain how the studies were appraised?

　　6. Is it possible to effectively compare the studies selected?

b) What are the results?

　　7. What do the results of the review mean?

　　8. How accurate are the results?

c) Will the results help my patients/clients care?

　　9. Are the results applicable to practice?

　　10. Are recommendations for practice made?

　　11. Should practice be changed as a result of this review?

Source: Adapted from Oxman *et al.* (1994).

are, what are the results? and (3) will the results help in my patient/client care? Each of these sections is further broken down to look at the research in more detail. Altogether there are 11 questions to answer. The first two questions are considered to be primary guides as they are useful in quickly screening out unsuitable studies. The other nine questions make up the secondary guide allowing a more thorough examination of the study to take place. As this is essentially a checklist, it is expected that you will end up with a list of 'yes', 'no' or 'cannot tell' answers. See Box 11.5 for a list of questions to ask about systematic reviews.

The difficulty with giving one word answers to these questions is that too many 'nos' or 'cannot tells' may cause you to struggle in deciding whether the study is valid. This illustrates the need to make explicit how you made your judgements when undertaking the appraisal. Your decisions will be subjective and a 'yes' or 'no' answer will not explain the thinking behind your decision. It is expected that the author of the systematic review will be explicit about the process that was used so it only seems fair that the person appraising the study is also explicit about the decision process that they went through. However, even if you decide following appraisal that it is a high-quality study, you need to remember that clinical experience and patient/client preferences may rule out the results. In Chapter 8, a definition of evidence-based nursing was explored which highlighted the importance of clinical expertise and patient/client preferences in making decisions about patient/client care (Di Censo *et al.* 1998). We must always have these issues on our mind when we are appraising any evidence, not just evidence provided by systematic reviews.

11.14 Conclusion

This chapter has introduced you to the concepts and skills necessary to search, critique and appraise evidence in a systematic way. It has identified stages of a literature search strategy and introduced you to the skills of critical thinking which are essential prerequisites to fulfil an effective appraisal. It has also highlighted that appraisal must take place once evidence has been selected but before it is put into practice. Appraisal is essential to ensuring that the evidence that we use in practice is good enough for the purpose that we want it. In addition, it needs to be applicable to the patient/client's needs and be suitable for use in the particular practice setting where we are working. Evidence on its own, however good, is of no use if it is not considered within the context of clinical expertise and patient/client preferences. It is recognized that evidence comes in many forms from research studies to clinical guidelines. In order to effectively appraise the variety of evidence that is available to us it is useful to have a framework or checklist to assist this often challenging process. Critical thinking and appraisal skills need to be learned and practised to have the desired effect. They are skills that you will need to develop as they are essential for contemporary nursing practice.

SELF-EVALUATION

? And, finally, your chance to revise what you have learnt from this chapter

- List the steps in the evidence-based practice process.

- Write out the seven stages of a literature search strategy.

- How would you describe the characteristics of critical thinking?

- What is the purpose of appraising clinical evidence?

- What are the pros and cons for clinicians of basing their practice on current best evidence?

- Why do we need to appraise the evidence instead of believing the abstract?

- What are the five areas to consider when appraising a research study?

- What appraisal tools are available for appraising research studies?

- Which tools could you use to appraise qualitative research?

- How would you appraise clinical guidelines?

- Which framework would you use to appraise a systematic review?

References

AGREE Collaboration (2003) Development and validation of an International appraisal instrument for assessing the quality of clinical practice guidelines: The AGREE project. *Quality and Safety in Health Care* 12: 18–23.

Boulton, M. and Fitzpatrick, R. (1997) Evaluating qualitative research. *Evidence-Based Health Policy and Management* 1(4): 83–85.

Burns, N. and Grove, S. (1987) *The Practice of Nursing Research: Conduct, Critique and Utilisation.* WB Saunders Company, Philadelphia.

Burns, N. and Grove, S. (1997) *The Practice of Nursing Research: Conduct, Critique and Utilisation* (Third edition). WB Saunders Company, Philadelphia.

Bury, T. and Jerosch-Herold, C. (1998) Reading and critical appraisal of the literature. In: Bury, T. and Mead, M. (eds) *Evidence-Based Healthcare: A Practical Guide for Therapists.* Butterworth-Heinemann, Oxford.

Case, B. (1994) Walking around the elephant: A critical thinking strategy for decision making. *Journal of Continuing Education in Nursing* 25(3): 101–109.

Cochrane Library (2003) *Issue 4.* Wiley and Sons Ltd, Chichester.

Critical Appraisal Skills Programme (CASP) (2002) 10 questions to help you make sense of qualitative research. Public Health Resource Unit, Milton Keynes.

Crombie, I. (1996) *The Pocket Guide to Critical Appraisal.* BMJ Publishing Group, London.

Cutcliffe, J. and Ward, M. (2003) *Critiquing Nursing Research.* Quay Books, Wiltshire.

De Poy, E. and Giltin, L.N. (1998) *Introduction to Research: Understanding and Applying Multiple Strategies.* St Louis, Mosby.

Di Censo, A., Cullum, N., and Ciliska, D. (1998) Implementing evidence-based nursing: Some misconceptions. *Evidence-Based Nursing* 1(2): 38–40.

Dixon, R., Munro, J., and Silcocks, P. (1997) *The Evidence-Based Medicine Workbook. Critical Appraisal for Clinical Problem Solving*. Butterworth-Heinemann, Oxford.

Duffy, M. (1985) A research appraisal checklist for evaluating nursing research reports. *Nursing Health Care* 6(10): 539–547.

Garratt, J., Overton, T., Tomlinson, J., and Clow, D. (2000) Critical thinking exercises for chemists: Are they subject specific? *Active Learning in Higher Education* 1(2): 152–167.

Greenlaugh, T. (2001) *How to Read a Research Paper. The Basics of Evidence Based Medicine*. BMJ Books, London.

Hill, A. and Spittlehouse, C. (2003) *What is Critical Appraisal?* Hayward Medical Communications, London.

Holloway, I. and Wheeler, S. (1996) *Qualitative Research for Nurses*. Blackwell Science, Oxford.

Hutchinson, A. and Baker, R. (1999) *Guidelines in Clinical Practice*. Radcliffe Medical Press, London.

Leininger, M. (1994) Evaluation criteria and critique of qualitative research studies. In: Morse, J. (ed.) *Critical Issues in Qualitative Research Methods*. Sage, California.

Le May, A. (1999) *Evidence-Based Practice*. Nursing Times Clinical Monographs No 1. NT Books, London.

Long, A. (2002) Critically appraising research studies. In: McSherry, R., Simmons, M., and Abbott, P. (eds) *Evidence-Informed Nursing: A Guide for Clinical Nurses*. Routledge, London.

Morrison, P. (1991) Critiquing research. *Surgical Nurse* 3(1): 20–22.

Newman, M. and Roberts, T. (2002) Critical appraisal I: Is the quality of the study good enough for you to use the findings? In: Craig, M. and Smyth, R. (eds) *The Evidence-Based Practice Manual for Nurses*. Churchill Livingstone, London.

NHS Centre for Reviews and Dissemination (1994) Implementing clinical practice guidelines: Can guidelines be used to improve clinical practice? *Effective Health Care* 1(18): 1–12.

Oxman, A., Cook, D., and Guyatt, G. (1994) Users' guides to the medical literature. VI. How to use an overview. *Journal of the American Medical Association* 272(17): 1367–1371.

Polit, D. and Beck, C. (2004) *Nursing Research: Principles and Methods*. Lippincott, Philadelphia.

Polit, D. and Hungler, B. (1997) *Essentials of Nursing Research: Methods, Appraisal and Utilisation* (Fourth edition). Lippincott, Philadelphia.

Popay, J. and Williams, G. (1998) Qualitative research and evidence-based health care. *Journal of the Royal Society of Medicine* 91 (Suppl 35): 32–37.

Royal College of Nursing (1996) *Clinical Effectiveness*. A Royal College of Nursing guide. Royal College of Nursing, London.

Seers, K. (2005) Qualitative research. In: Dawes, M., Davies, P., Gray, A., Mant, J., Seers, K., and Snowball, R. (eds) *Evidence-Based Practice: A Primer for Health Care Professionals*. Elsevier Churchill Livingstone, London.

Snowball, R. (2005). Critical appraisal of clinical practice guidelines. In: Dawes, M., Davies, P., Gray, A., Mant, J., Seers, K., and Snowball, R. (eds) *Evidence-Based Practice: A Primer for Health Care Professionals*. Elsevier Churchill Livingstone, London.

Spencer, L., Ritchie, J., Lewis, J., and Dillon, L. (2003) *Quality in Qualitative Evaluation: A Framework for Assessing Research Evidence*. National Centre for Social Research. Occasional papers series 2. Government Chief Social Researcher's Office, Cabinet Office, London.

Strauss, A. and Corbin, J. (1990) *Basics of Qualitative Research: Grounded Theory Procedures and Techniques*. Sage, California.

Thompson, C. (1999) Searching for the evidence. *Nursing Times Learning Curve* 3(3): 12–13.

Thompson, C. and Cullum, N. (1999) Examining the evidence: An overview. *Nursing Times Learning Curve* 1(3): 7–9.

@ Useful resources to explore critique and appraisal of evidence

Websites worth visiting

Appraising qualitative research
www.policyhub.gov.uk/evalpolicy/qual_eval.asp
www.phru.nhs.uk/casp/qualitat.htm

Appraising clinical guidelines
www.agreecollaboration.org

Appraising systematic reviews
www.phru.nhs.uk/casp/reviews.htm

Suggested reading

Cutcliffe, J. and Ward, M. (2003) *Critiquing Nursing Research*. Quay Books, Wiltshire.
   This book contains worked examples of four frameworks used to appraise research studies.
Ogier, M. and Lanoe, N. (2002) *Ogier's Reading Research*. Baillière Tindall, London.
   This is a step-by-step guide written in a down-to-earth manner to finding your way around research reports and deciding whether they are relevant to practice.
Polit, D. and Beck, C. (2003) *Nursing Research: Principles and Methods*. Lippincott, Philadelphia.
   This book provides an overview of most aspects of research that are related to nursing. It is a useful book to consult when you are unsure about research terms. The only thing to remember is that it is an American text and therefore may contain some anomalies.

12

Applying Knowledge to Practice

Andrée le May

CONTENTS

- Tacit and explicit knowledge
- Mechanisms for applying knowledge to practice
- Communities of Practice
- Knowledge Networks

LEARNING OUTCOMES

This chapter should enable you to

- Extend your knowledge about the types of knowledge that you and others use in practice and the value that you place on them
- Consider various mechanisms for applying knowledge to practice and their effectiveness in your day-to-day practice
- Think about situations where you could use Communities of Practice and Knowledge Networks to make your care better and your work more effective
- Think about how you will help others to apply knowledge and evaluate its effectiveness in the future.

12.1 Introduction

This book has shown how nurses have built up their knowledge over centuries of practice, theory development and research. The challenge for nurses, midwives and health visitors now, and well into the future, is not only generating knowledge for practice but also applying knowledge appropriately and creatively to practice. In order to do this successfully, nurses need to use all of the knowledge and skills referred to in the preceding chapters. Knowing where nursing has come from, its ethical values and where it is going to (Chapters 1–5) will help you to contextualize the development of knowledge for practice and understand some of the complexities around its application. This application of knowledge to practice is dependent not only on having the right knowledge to appraise and deliver effective care (Chapters 10 and 11) but also being able to lead and manage care skilfully (Chapters 8 and 9) within an ever-changing health and social care context (Chapters 6 and 7).

This final chapter further considers types of knowledge that underpin practice but in the context of how practitioners may apply such knowledge, either individually or collectively, in practice. This chapter challenges you to think about ways in which you might enhance your practice through the application of knowledge both now and in the future.

12.2 Tacit and explicit knowledge

In the first chapter of this book, Janice Brown and Mary Gobbi talked about various standards or codes of practice that explicitly set out the knowledge and skills that nurses need to have to become competent practitioners. This sort of knowledge is known as explicit knowledge since it is recorded and easily passed on between people ensuring that nurses are taught to a similar level, practice to an agreed standard and that their competence can be assessed in order to safeguard patients and the public. As nurses become more experienced, their knowledge base becomes more extensive and more complicated; their explicit knowledge gained from various sources becomes merged with experience to form a bricolage (Gobbi 2005) that, when used, best fits the immediate and often complex needs of practice. Over time, this explicit knowledge becomes deeply embedded in nurses' minds and is often hard to articulate and pass on to others – it is internalized and changes at this point from explicit to tacit knowledge.

Tacit knowledge, when it combines appropriate explicit and experiential knowledge, is greatly valued and often unique to individual nurses making them expert practitioners and opinion leaders in their area of practice. It is to these experts that more junior or less experienced practitioners often turn for knowledge and advice and the act of giving this advice makes their tacit knowledge explicit and transferable to others again. So in this way nursing knowledge becomes richer as it is passed on from one person to another.

ACTIVITY 12.1

Consider the sorts of knowledge that you use in practice – are they explicit or tacit? What is the difference between them in your experience?

12.3 Mechanisms for applying knowledge to practice

Using the best and most up-to-date knowledge appropriately for each nursing situation is one of the central tenets of effective practice. This, on the face of it, seems straightforward enough however, it often requires some kind of alteration to already established patterns of behaviour and as such is more difficult to achieve than it may first appear. In the 1990s, considerable effort was spent constructing ways to help practitioners to apply knowledge to practice in order to make care more effective and efficient. Most of these mechanisms focussed on packaging knowledge up in different ways and presenting it to practitioners with the expectation that they would then simply implement it: little attention was spent on trying to understand how people actually used knowledge in their practice and how, therefore, knowledge should be given to them to make implementation easier. Many of these mechanisms are still used to encourage the application of knowledge to practice today, with varying success. They include:

- Ongoing educational opportunities following qualification
- The use of guidelines to guide and change practice
- The use of local opinion leaders
- Audit and feedback
- Manual and computerized reminder systems.

(NHS CRD 1999)

ACTIVITY 12.2

List the various mechanisms for applying knowledge to practice that you have used in the last six months and think about their effectiveness in helping you to apply knowledge to your practice.

Despite a great deal of attention and resource being spent on these interventions during the last decade, there still remains a gap between the availability of knowledge and its application. The existence of this gap has led to the creation of several initiatives to raise the profile of evidence-based practice and the implementation of knowledge with the most ambitious probably being the creation of the Modernisation Agency (MA) under the NHS Plan (DoH 2000a). This agency was established in order to provide the NHS with a centre focussing on how knowledge and 'know how' about best practice could be spread (DoH 2000b). The MA, although now subsumed by the NHS Institute for Innovation and Improvement, presented many opportunities for networking, learning from and working alongside others in order to change practice and the development of leadership skills that would enable the implementation of knowledge and alteration of practice.

The new Institute will carry on offering opportunities for people to enhance practice by:

- Working closely with clinicians, NHS organizations, patients, the public, academia and industry in the UK and worldwide to identify best practice.

- Developing the NHS' capability for service transformation, technology and product innovation, leadership development and learning.

- Supporting the rapid adoption and spread of new ideas by providing guidance on practical change ideas and ways to facilitate local, safe implementation.

- Promoting a culture of innovation and life-long learning for all NHS staff.

In addition to these government initiatives, researchers are also trying to understand, often by observing practice, the sorts of knowledge that practitioners actually use on a day-to-day basis in order to deliver good care. This type of research is useful because it allows us to understand what really happens in practice and as a result of this to plan better ways for applying knowledge. Some recent ethnographic research by Gabbay and le May (2004, EBN 2005) suggests that practitioners in primary care rarely accessed and used explicit knowledge from research or other sources directly, but relied on 'mindlines' which were collectively reinforced, internalized, tacit sources of knowledge – or personal guidelines. Whilst these were informed by brief reading they were also affected by their own and their colleagues' experience, their interactions with each other and with opinion leaders, patients, pharmaceutical representatives and other sources of largely tacit knowledge. Influenced by organizational demands and constraints, mindlines were continuously negotiated, socially, with a variety of key people – predominantly patients and colleagues, resulting in knowledge appropriate for their practice. This research emphasizes the value of interaction in the process of knowledge application – testing out knowledge with colleagues and using their knowledge as well as one's own to inform practice; it also emphasizes the importance of merging knowledge from different sources (a little like the bricolage suggested by Gobbi 2005).

As a result of this, and other works, it is beginning to be recognized that the effective transfer of knowledge often takes place through people and not through the dissemination and reading of printed media such as guidelines, policies and research papers. This means that increased emphasis should be placed on finding ways by which people can get together to share knowledge about, and shape knowledge for, their practice. These interactions naturally facilitate the transformation of tacit knowledge into explicit knowledge and discussions related to the application of knowledge to practice. Two good examples of this kind of mechanism for encouraging the transfer and application of knowledge to practice are Communities of Practice and Knowledge Networks.

12.4 Communities of practice

Wenger, McDermott and Snyder (2001: 4/5) defined Communities of Practice as '... groups of people who share a concern, a set of problems, or a passion about a topic, and who deepen their understanding and knowledge of this area by interacting on an ongoing basis.... These people don't necessarily work together on a day-to-day basis, but they get together because they find value in their interactions. As they spend time together, they typically share information, insight, and advice. They solve problems. They help each other. They discuss their situation, their aspirations, their needs. They think about common issues. They explore ideas and act as sounding boards to each other. They may create tools, standards, generic designs, manuals, and other documents; or they may just keep what they know as a tacit understanding they share.... Over time, they develop a unique perspective on their topic as well as a body of common knowledge, practices, and approaches. They also develop personal relationships and established ways of interacting. They may even develop a common sense of identity. They become a community of practice.'

Increasingly, Communities of Practice are forming in health and social care settings as one means of developing best practice, implementing new knowledge or shaping old knowledge for new practices in order that people might do their jobs better on a day-to-day basis. Communities of Practice are ideal mechanisms through which people can discuss the best ways to implement knowledge to suit the needs and context of their area of practice or particular patients. They can function either as 'real' face-to-face communities or virtually via interactive learning environments or electronic discussion groups. To be effective, Communities of Practice need to pay attention to:

- *Membership* in terms of who is chosen to be involved initially and throughout the life of the Community of Practice, the extent (active or passive) and legitimacy of their involvement, their knowledge base and expertise, and the importance of their involvement to achieving the goal of the group and the alterations planned to care/services.

- *Commitment* from *within* the community to the desired goals and from *outside* the community in order to develop any required service/practice alterations.

- *Relevance* to local communities and the existing services/professional groups/groups of patients to enable acceptance of the change.

- *Enthusiasm* that could be personal, professional or service-related for the area being considered by the Community of Practice.

- *Infrastructure* to support the work of the Community of Practice in terms of ease of access to knowledge or evidence (e.g. availability of library resources and information technology, particular experts or opinion leaders) and resources which are available in order to find information about current services (e.g. networks, statistics, documents).

■ *Skills* in relation to accessing and appraising a variety of sources of knowledge together with those needed in bringing evidence together into a coherent plan for action by the Community of Practice. For instance, this might involve writing action plans, reports or business plans.

■ *Resources* for achieving the desired change that go beyond the time needed to meet, seek information or canvas support. These could include pump-priming money for pilot work in relation to the desired service change or funds for evaluating the effects of change on the quality of care provided by the new service.

(Adapted from Lathlean and le May 2002)

Communities of Practice are beneficial not only for the people who form them, but also for the organizations within which, or across which, they function since they are very powerful ways for sharing and applying knowledge whilst motivating participants to improve care. They therefore have the potential to positively impact on the:

■ Standard of care delivered to patients

■ Working environments and job satisfaction of the participants in the Community

■ Speed with which day-to-day problems are solved

■ Speed with which knowledge and innovation moves into practice

■ Creation of a unified team which may be uni- or multi-professional

■ Ownership and sustainability of changes to practice.

ACTIVITY 12.3

Think of a situation/issue around which you might develop a Community of Practice as a means of enhancing care. How would you go about this?

12.5 Knowledge networks

There is increasing interest in developing knowledge sharing networks that enable knowledge to be passed on within and between organizations. These are often groups of experts who work together to share knowledge and solve challenges that are of interest to the membership of the networks. These networks range from small groups of individuals, perhaps working in Communities of

Practice, to larger regionally or nationally based networks formed from different professional groups who share a common interest (e.g. the NHS Cancer Research Network [NCRN] and the newly created Diabetes Networks).

These networks can be built around exisitng organizational structures (e.g. special interest groups in professional organizations, for instance the Royal College of Nursing's professional forums and groups) or social networks of people informally drawn together as a result of common interests and enthusiasms. They traditionally provide access to information and also people with expertise and knowledge. Their increasing popularity is due perhaps to claims that they 'enable participants (to) constantly shape and extend the activities of these networks in response to real needs and challenges' (Cukor and McKnight 2001: 4), so they are very much about solving day-to-day problems and passing on knowledge which would be immediately useful to practice.

Some of the attractions of belonging to such a network include:

- Having quick and easy access to people who might be able to give answers to practice-related questions

- Providing an opportunity to 'network' with others who share the same area of interest and may be like-minded

- Having a platform from which to influence others at a local and/or national level

- Being able to contact experts whose opinion you trust (probably because you are a member of the same network)

- Being able to learn from others.

ACTIVITY 12.4

Identify a Knowledge Network in your unit/directorate and map out its members and their expertise. Ask two of them about its value in their day-to-day practice.

12.6 Conclusions

Nurses around the world have been basing their practice on knowledge, from a variety of sources, since the creation of their respective roles. Originally, the knowledge that supported practice was linked to other professions' knowledge bases, experience and guidance; now, however, nurses are more able to use their own sources of knowledge, uniquely shaped to their professional responsibilities and increasingly developed from and informed by research. The evidence-based practice movement has been, and continues to be, strongly supported by governmental, professional and individual demands for effective care based on appropriate and identifiable knowledge/evidence, together with the evaluation of the impact of that knowledge through audit and further research. Clinical guidelines, care pathways and the use of systematic reviews of literature are some examples of the increasing variety of guidance developed to direct and standardize practice; whilst formal mechanisms for evaluating the quality of care provide a strong impetus to ensure the appropriate use of knowledge within many different practice scenarios. The really hard part of applying knowledge to practice is working with people to improve collaboration and knowledge sharing.

Some of the challenges for twenty-first century nurses revolve around:

■ Working collaboratively with colleagues and patients to ensure that the best knowledge is applied in practice in order to deliver the best possible care.

■ Understanding how, in a variety of practice situations, knowledge is shaped and its application negotiated between practitioners and individual patients, groups of patients or communities.

■ Developing mechanisms for re-embedding knowledge shaped by practice back into our professional knowledge base so that it becomes richer and deeper.

■ Determining if particular types of knowledge provide a firmer foundation upon which practice can be built and updated than others.

SELF-EVALUATION

And, finally, your chance to revise what you have learnt from this chapter

■ What is the difference between tacit and explicit knowledge?

■ What are Communities of Practice and how might they help knowledge to be applied to practice?

■ What sorts of Knowledge Networks do you have access to?

■ How will you help others to apply knowledge and evaluate its effectiveness in the future?

References

Cukor, P. and McKnight, L. (2001) *Knowledge Networks, the Internet and Development.* Tufts University, Boston.

Department of Health (DoH) (2000a) *The NHS Plan: A Plan for Investment, a Plan for Reform.* DH, London.

Department of Health (DoH) (2000b) *The NHS Plan: Implementing the Performance Improvement Agenda. A Policy Position Statement and Consultation Document.* DH, London.

Evidence-Based Nursing (EBN) (2005) Primary care practitioners based everyday practice on internalised tacit guidelines derived through social interactions with trusted colleagues. *EBN* 8: 94.

Gabbay, J. and le May, A. (2004) Evidence-based guidelines or collectively constructed 'mind-lines'? An ethnographic study of knowledge management in primary care. *British Medical Journal* 329 (October 30) 1013–1016.

Gobbi, M. (2005) Nursing practice as bricoleur activity: A concept explored. *Nursing Inquiry* 12(2): 17–125.

Lathlean, J. and le May, A. (2002) Communities of Practice – an opportunity for inter-agency working. *Journal of Clinical Nursing* 11: 394–398.

NHS Centre for Reviews and Dissemination (1999) Getting evidence into practice. *Effective Health Care* 5(1): 1–16, University of York.

Wenger, E., McDermott, R., and Snyder, W. (2001) *Cultivating Communities of Practice*. Harvard Business School, Harvard.

Suggested reading

Wenger, E., McDermott, R., and Snyder, W. (2001) *Cultivating Communities of Practice*. Harvard Business School, Harvard.

This book defines the unique features of Communities of Practice and outlines principles of their essential elements. It provides guidelines to support Communities of Practice through their major stages of development, addresses the potential downsides of Communities, and discusses the specific challenges of distributed communities.

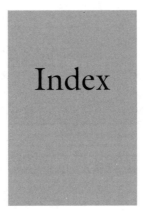

Index